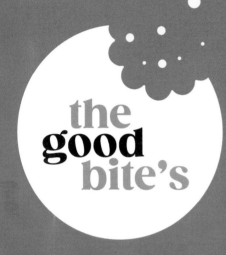

the good bite's
High Protein
MEAL PREP MANUAL

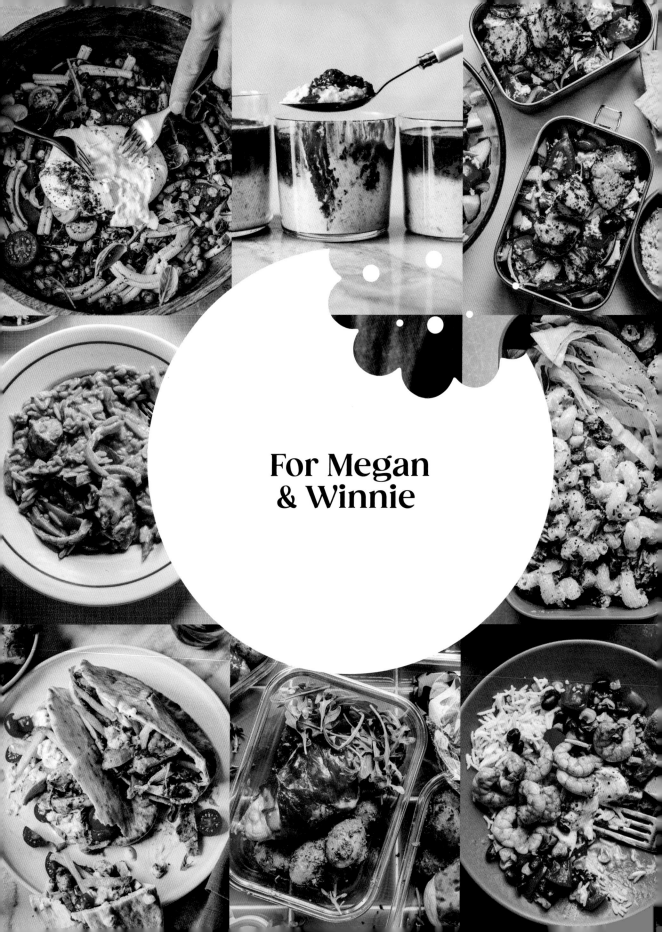

For Megan
& Winnie

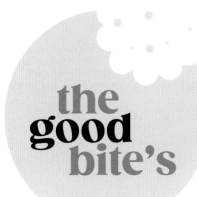

the good bite's

High Protein

MEAL PREP MANUAL

Niall Kirkland

**Delicious, easy, low-calorie recipes
with full nutritional breakdowns
and food-tracking barcodes**

Photography by
HAARALA HAMILTON

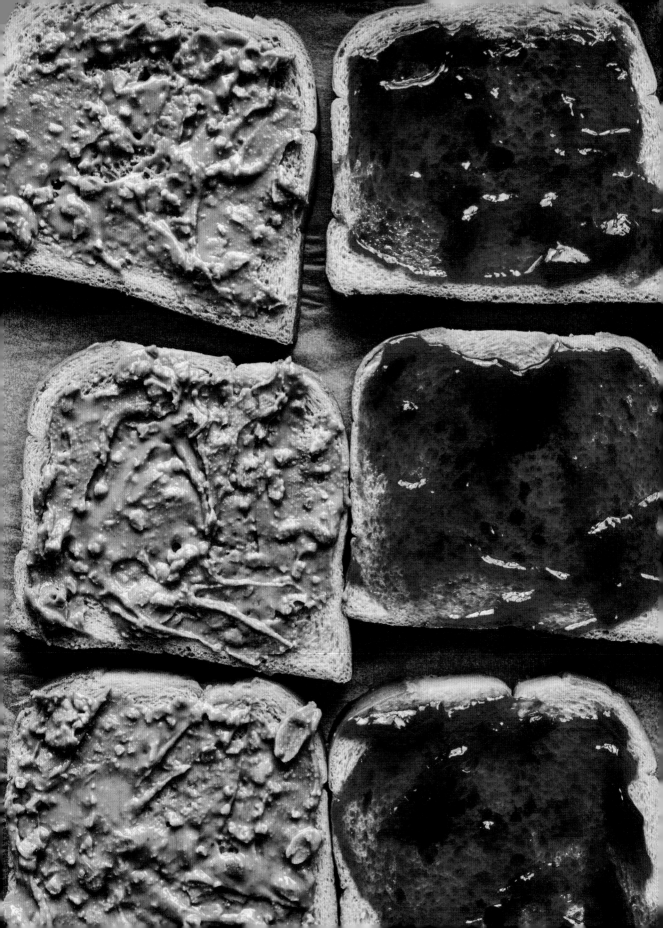

Contents

Welcome

Welcome to
The Good Bite...

I truly believe that a healthy lifestyle goes hand in hand with delicious food. If you make meals that are fun, tasty and interesting, with twists on the classics and sweet treats that satisfy your sweet tooth, while making a positive impact on your health, then you will eat well and feel great in yourself, every single day. And that's the important part. If you truly love what you are eating, then your diet will be sustainable and when you are consistent, you get great results. Good food, good feels!

My name is Niall Kirkland, I'm a recipe creator and I've made it my mission to find a more joyful, easy way to eat healthy, high-protein meals. My recipes aim to take away the stress of not knowing which ingredients will give you what nutritionally and how to combine them to get the most out of your mealtimes. Included are nutritionist-approved calorie, carbohydrate, protein and fat breakdowns for each recipe, along with barcodes so you can scan meals straight into your food diary app. What is a good bite to me? – the perfect balance of easy, healthy and completely mouth-watering. This cookbook is my first bound collection of the very best of them and I'm so excited to share them with you.

Just over two years ago I set up The Good Bite. Ever since then, I haven't been able to stop writing and developing healthy, delicious meals for my followers. With a passion for both fitness and food, I wanted to provide people with easy ways to eat what they love while getting all the nutrition they need to lead a healthy and active lifestyle. I wanted to focus on meal prep for this book because I believe it to be one of the most vital parts of keeping yourself on track. How often do we reach for the takeaway menu or a quick, unhealthy fix when we are tired and hungry and there's nothing ready to eat in the fridge? You'll notice from this book that I don't believe in completely restricting any types of foods from my diet. I love eating pasta, bread and chocolate for instance, foods that have been labelled as 'bad' over the years, but I believe that you can fit all of these foods in your diet as long as you're holding yourself accountable and eating them within moderation. I've done the thinking for you with this book by creating recipes with generous portion sizes and modest calorie counts. A focus on high protein has meant that I have been able to add food to my diet instead of removing it. Ingredients like chicken, beef, tuna, salmon, eggs, almonds, oats, black beans, lentils, cheese and yoghurt are just some of the produce available on the high-protein menu. With ingredients like this, I knew I could create some really generous, hearty meals. So often doing without is what we associate with healthy eating, but *The Good Bite* will show you that simply isn't true. You can enjoy what you love. Inside *The Good Bite's High Protein, Meal Prep Manual* you'll find 80 recipes that harness the power of protein to complement an active lifestyle, all while tasting really indulgent.

If you get the small stuff right then everything else falls into place. The recipes inside this book are fuss-free, easy to cook and contain accessible ingredients all found in your local supermarket – some you might already have in your cupboard at home too. Inside this cookbook you'll find one-pot meals so you can add your ingredients to one pan, pot or baking dish and let your cooker or slow cooker do the hard work for you. Others are super speedy for when you're in a hurry on a busy weeknight. Lots are low in calories and are perfect for anyone who is on a weight-loss journey. Some recipes make the most of your air fryer for speed, low fat, amazing crunchy texture and will save on your energy bills. All of the recipes inside are perfect for meal prepping so you can cook once, fill your fridge with tasty feasts and eat good food all week long.

I really hope you love cooking the recipes in this book as much as I have loved creating (and eating) them.

Niall x

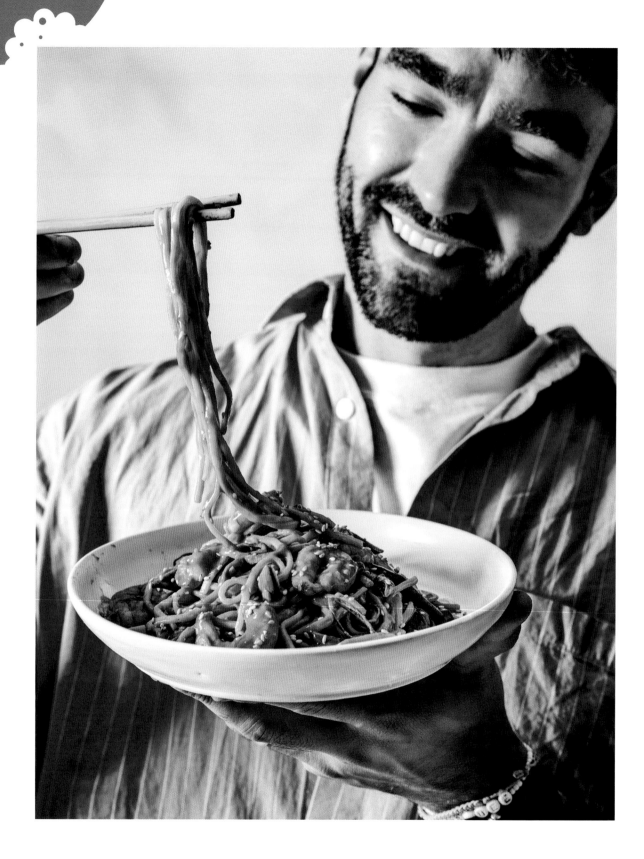

Why Eat a Protein-rich Diet?

Protein isn't exclusively for fitness fanatics. Eating high protein has benefits for everyone who wants to support a healthy, active lifestyle, no matter your fitness goal. Let me fill you in on the important rewards of eating protein-rich meals.

1. Foods that are high in protein will sustain your appetite for much longer. It'll banish that 3 p.m. Monday afternoon all-consuming want-to-snack feeling. Protein-rich meals take longer to break down compared to fatty and carbohydrate-heavy foods, so they will keep you feeling fuller for longer. Protein also lowers Ghrelin levels – your hunger hormone. So, if you are trying to lose some weight through consuming fewer calories, eating protein is the effortless way to having more control over your appetite without trying to eat much less than you do already.

2. Eating more protein will help your body recover faster from exercise; it will do wonders for your overall health, the strength of your bones and keeps age-related muscle loss at bay. Eating protein gives us the building blocks for essential functions like the growth of cells and tissue, and it is great for our immunity too.

Protein is your go-to superfood that works for your body like no other superfood. And the best thing? It's cost-effective and available everywhere.

How Much Protein Should I Be Aiming For?

We can work out our own recommended daily amount of protein based on how much we need per kilogram (kg) of our bodyweight. For adults this is 0.8g per kg of our bodyweight. On average it is recommended that women (based on a 60kg bodyweight) have 48g of protein per day. On average for men (based on a 75kg bodyweight) it is 60g of protein per day. To build lean muscle your protein intake can be more than the average stated above. Studies have shown that higher protein intakes of 1.5g per kg of bodyweight daily, alongside resistance weight training, works for optimum muscle strength and building. I recommend speaking to a qualified nutritionist before attempting to increase your protein intake from the recommended average.

Here is a chart of protein content for common ingredients:

Ingredient	Protein content (g) per 100g/100ml	Ingredient	Protein content (g) per 100g/100ml
Chicken breast (grilled)	32g	Semi-skimmed milk	3.5g
Beef steak	31g	Oat milk	1.1g
Lamb chop	29.2g	Almond milk	1.3g
Pork chop	31.6g	Red lentils (boiled)	7.6g
Cod (baked)	23.9g	Chickpeas (tinned)	6.7g
Salmon (grilled)	24.6g	Black beans (tinned)	8.9g
Tuna (tinned)	24.9g	Kidney beans (tinned)	6.9g
Prawns	15.4g	Baked beans	5g
Egg (boiled)	14.1g	Almonds	29g
Plain low-fat yoghurt	4.8g	Hazelnuts	14.1g
Plain Greek-style yoghurt	5.7g	Walnuts	15g
Cottage cheese	9.4g	Rice (boiled)	8.2g
Cheddar cheese	25.4g	Pasta (boiled)	5.7g
Reduced-fat Cheddar	27.9g	Porridge oats	11.1g
Whole milk	3.4g	Brown bread	7.9g
		White bread	7.9g
		Tofu	8.1g
		Tempeh	19g

How the Recipes Work

What is a Good Bite? Healthy? Of course. High protein? Most definitely. But, above all, DELICIOUS! I don't hold with the idea that healthy food should leave you wanting more or feeling less satisfied, and I've always been on a mission to bridge the gap between nutritious and delicious. The recipes in this book serve four people, so you can feed your family and friends easily. They are divided into nine tasty chapters, covering Breakfast Bites (page 16); Hot, Hot, Hot Lunches (page 36); Sandwiches & Salads (page 60); Perfect Pastas (page 78); Noodles & Rice (page 98); Weeknight Feasts (page 124); Favourite Fakeaways (page 140); Set & Forget Slow Cooks (page 162); and Protein Puds (page 178). Within those chapters you'll find high-protein versions of all your favourite meals, each one packed with flavour and nutritionally balanced so that they're as kind to your body as they are to your tastebuds. Curries, pies, burgers, ramen, fried chicken, toasties, lasagne, even cheesecake! You name it, we've got it!

Nutritional Info and Recipe Barcodes

For each recipe you'll find a full nutritional breakdown, making it easy to identify protein, calories, carbs and fat, so that you can easily keep track and make sure you're hitting the targets for all your macros. For those who use MyFitnessPal or Nutracheck, each recipe includes a barcode that can be scanned directly into the app so that you can keep on top of your daily targets.

Light Bites

For those on a weight-loss journey, or who are just looking to eat something on the lighter side, recipes labelled as 'light bites' are those with 500 calories or less. There is an easy-to-spot symbol on the top of each light bite recipe.

Air Fryer and Slow Cooker Recipes

It's no secret that air fryers and slow cookers are at the top of everyone's Christmas list at the moment, and it's no wonder. They're energy efficient and can save you time and money. You'll find a whole chapter of set-and-forget slow cooker recipes on page 162 and for recipes that can be prepared in an air fryer, we've included air fryer symbols.

Quick Bites

When you need healthy, delicious meals and fast, these quick recipes are cooked in 20 minutes or under and are perfect for slotting into your week no matter what your plans are. Like your light bites, these are easy to find with a symbol marking each one.

Veggie Bites

For your Meat-Free Mondays or any time in the week you'd like to increase your veggie intake there are high protein vegetarian recipes marked with this symbol.

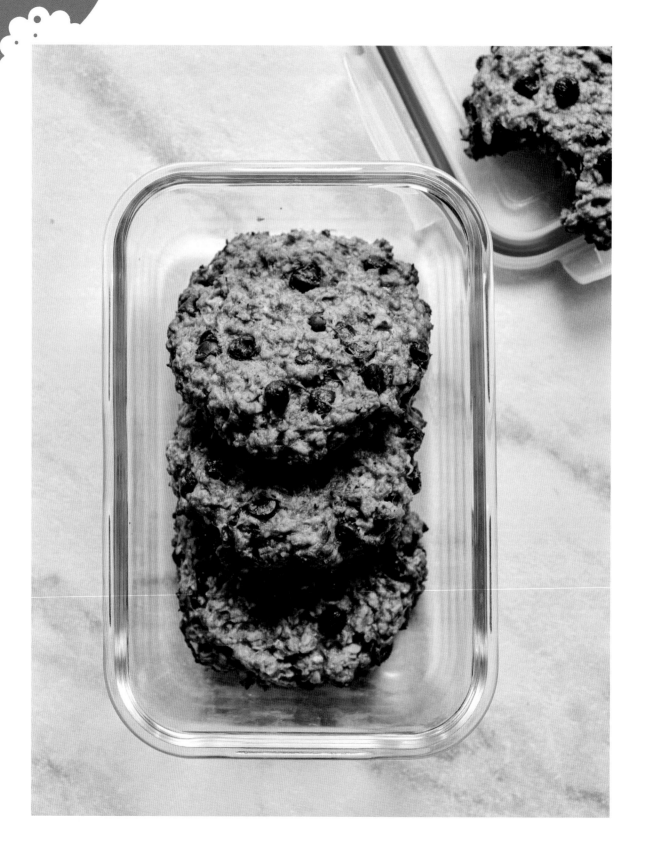

The Magic of Meal Prep

We've all been there. You get home from work at the end of a long day, stare half-heartedly into a sad, almost-empty fridge for inspiration, slump on the sofa and reach for your phone to scroll through your favourite meal delivery app. Recognise this picture? Meal prep is the answer!

Allocating a couple of hours at the weekend or on a quiet evening in the week to fill your fridge with delicious, healthy, high-protein meals that will eliminate the temptation of takeaway and take all of the stress out of knowing what to eat in the evening is a sure-fire way to save you time, money and keep you eating nutritious meals all week long.

For the most part, the recipes in this book are designed to feed about four people, but portioned up and kept in the fridge they can feed a single person over four nights or a couple over two. All of these recipes will keep well in the fridge for 3–4 days, and I've included easy instructions for reheating and bringing them back to life so that they're just as enjoyable on day three or four as they are on day one.

For your prepped meals, make sure they are stored in airtight containers or they are well wrapped in tin foil or cling film. Put them into the fridge as soon as you can after cooking. Reheat your meals in the air fryer at 180°C for up to 10 minutes or until heated all the way through. In the oven, preheat to 200°C and cook for up to 20 minutes, or until heated all the way through.

I'm generally cooking for just Megan and myself so I tend to make a couple of meals on a Sunday evening that will keep us both fed for the week. Doing it this way means that you can alternate the meals from day to day, so that it never feels repetitive. Keeping one day free gives you a bit of flexibility, if you fancy a meal out or the call of a takeaway pizza is too much to ignore. Be realistic and plan for your own lifestyle – there's no right or wrong way to do this!

I don't just meal prep for evening meals, and in the pages of this book you'll find delicious breakfasts, snacks, sweet treats and light lunches, all of which can be made ahead and stored in the same way, so your fridge is always bursting with vibrant, satisfying options to keep you on track with your goals, whether they are to support training, weight loss or just to eat delicious food. We've got you covered!

Aside from having delicious and nutritious food at your fingertips, planning and cooking your meals like this is also a brilliant way of saving money and reducing waste. Plan your meals, write your shopping list and stick to it when you go to the shops. You'll be amazed at how quickly your food bills go down. By only buying food that you know you're actually going to eat, you won't be spending your hard-earned cash on food that will be thrown away uneaten a week later, which is far better for both your wallet and the planet. Win, win!

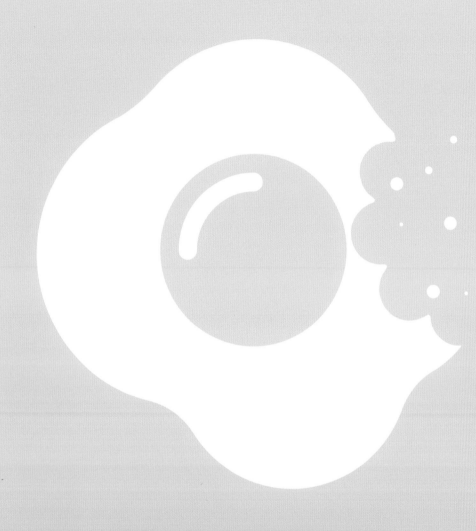

Breakfast
Bites

Sausage, Spicy Egg & Cheese Muffins

Everybody loves a breakfast muffin, so save yourself money and a trip to the drive-thru by making these! They are delicious, full of flavour (with a hint of spice from the fresh jalapeño) and absolutely perfect for prepping ahead.

6 eggs
25ml semi-skimmed milk
1 fresh jalapeño, deseeded and finely chopped
a handful of fresh chives, chopped
10 low-fat chicken sausages
½ tsp smoked paprika
½ tsp garlic granules
4 English muffins, sliced in half
2 tbsp light cream cheese
ketchup (optional)
4 American cheese slices
low-calorie cooking spray
salt and freshly ground black pepper

1. Preheat the oven to 200°C (180°C fan/400°F/Gas 6) and spray a baking dish with low-calorie cooking spray.

2. In a bowl, whisk together the eggs, milk, jalapeño and chives and season with salt and pepper. Transfer to the prepared baking dish and bake for 8–10 minutes, stirring halfway through, until cooked. Slice the baked egg into four pieces and remove from the baking dish.

3. Remove the sausages from their skins, place the sausage meat in a bowl, then mix with the smoked paprika and garlic granules. Form into four patties. Pack the sausage mixture into circle moulds, if you have them, or else shape into rounds, then transfer to an air fryer basket or large, non-stick frying pan and spray all over with low-calorie cooking spray.

4. Cook in the air fryer at 200°C for 5–7 minutes until cooked through or pan-fry for 3–4 minutes on each side.

5. Lightly toast the English muffins, then spread the cream cheese on the bottom slices and ketchup on the top slices, if using. Stack the muffins with the sausage patties, cheese slices and then baked egg slices.

6. Store in an airtight container in the fridge for up to 3 days, wrap in tin foil or put in an air-tight freezer bag and freeze for up to 3 months.

Protein
31.8g

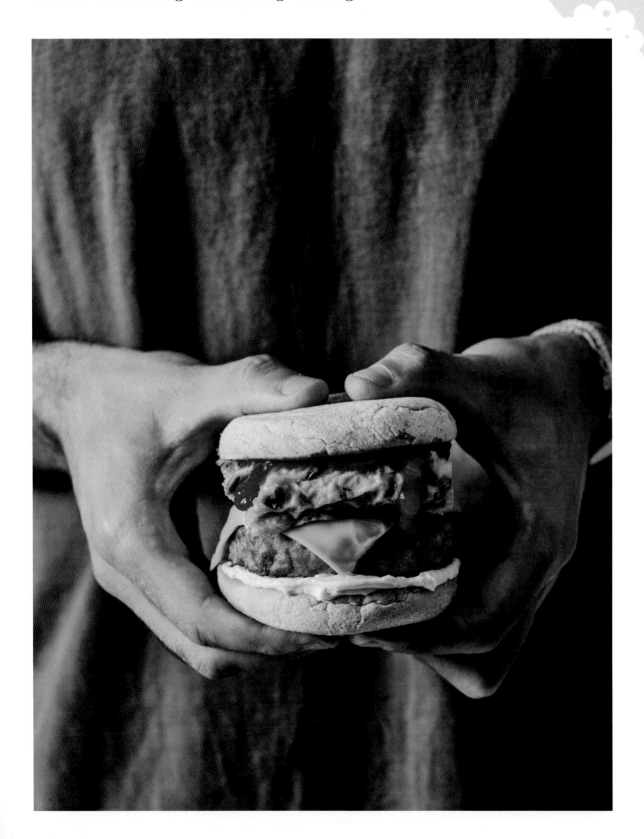

Garlic & Herb Frittata Bagel

These frittata bagels are the perfect on-the-go, high-protein breakfast option. A tasty, oven baked frittata is sliced and packed into a seeded bagel with garlic and herb cream cheese. Store these in the fridge or freezer and they'll reheat perfectly when you need them.

4 eggs
4 egg whites
2 handfuls of spinach, chopped
a handful of fresh basil, chopped
1 sweet Romano pepper,
 finely chopped
4 lean bacon medallions,
 thinly sliced
a pinch of chilli flakes
4 tbsp Boursin or garlic and herb
 cream cheese
4 seeded bagels, sliced in half
low-calorie cooking spray
salt and freshly ground
 black pepper

1. Preheat the oven to 200°C (180°C fan/400°F/Gas 6) and spray a baking dish with low-calorie cooking spray.

2. Put the eggs, egg whites, spinach, basil, Romano pepper, bacon medallions and chilli flakes into a large bowl, season with salt and pepper and mix until combined. Transfer the egg mixture to the prepared baking dish and bake for 12–15 minutes until cooked through.

3. Remove from the oven and slice the frittata into four pieces (or, if you used a bigger dish and the frittata is thinner, double up and slice into eight pieces). Lightly toast the bagels and spread the Boursin or cream cheese onto both sides, then use them to sandwich the frittata slices.

4. Transfer to an airtight container or wrap in tin foil and store in the fridge for up to 3 days. Freeze in an airtight freezer bag for up to 3 months.

Protein
28.8g

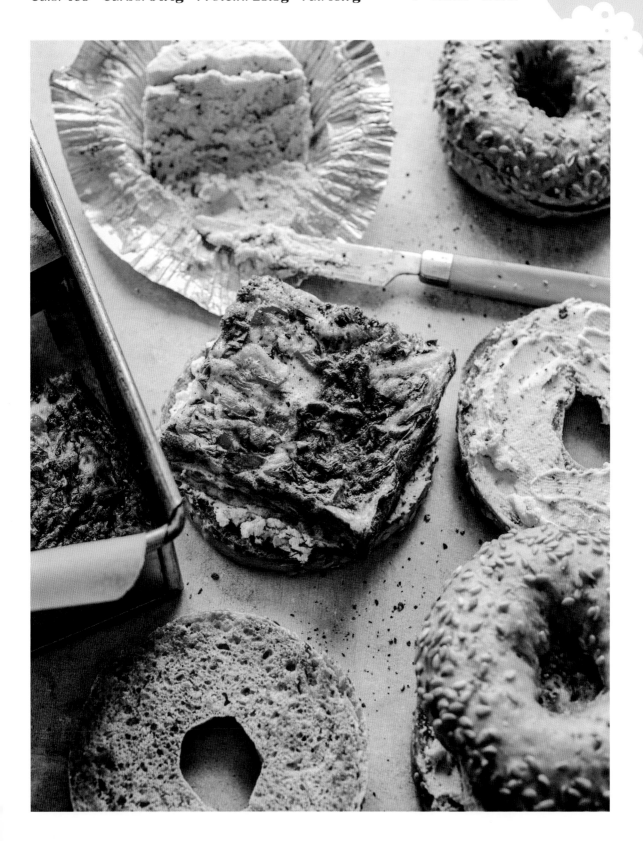

Serves: **4**   Prep time: **5 mins**   Cook time: **10 mins**

Cals: **539**   Carbs: **38.4g**   Protein: **28.6g**   Fat: **30.7g**

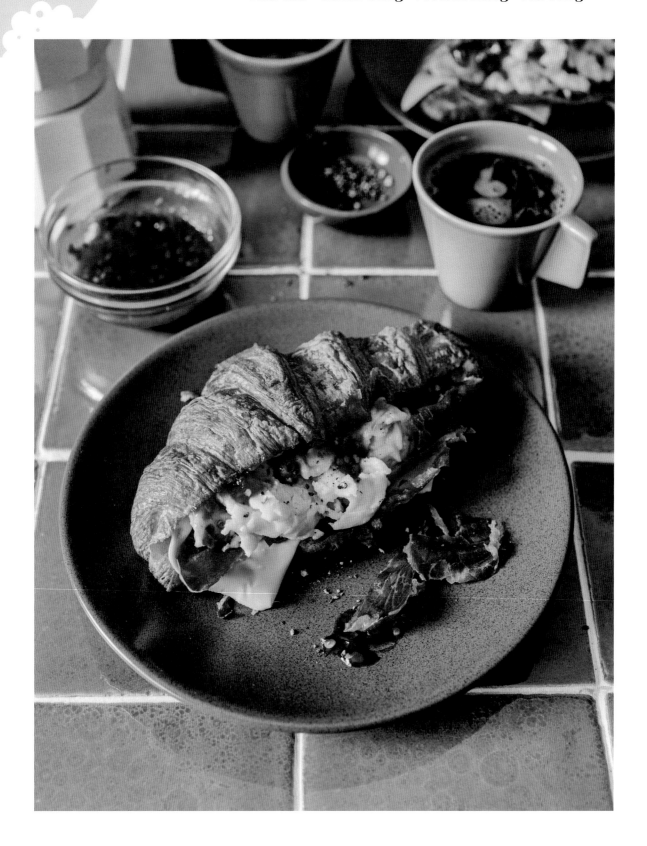

Make-ahead Breakfast Croissants

Crispy prosciutto, soft scrambled eggs, cheese and chilli jam make these savoury breakfast croissants a delicious make-ahead breakfast for the week. They crisp up perfectly when reheated in an oven or an air fryer. Best served hot.

8 slices of prosciutto
6 eggs
4 croissants, sliced open
4 American cheese slices, sliced in
   half diagonally
4 tbsp chilli jam
low-calorie cooking spray
salt and freshly ground
   black pepper

1. Preheat the oven to 200°C (180°C fan/400°F/Gas 6) and line a baking tray with baking paper.

2. Lay the prosciutto out on the prepared baking tray and bake in the oven for 5–6 minutes until crisp. Alternatively, cook in an air fryer in two batches at 200°C for 3–4 minutes.

3. Meanwhile, whisk the eggs in a bowl and season with salt and pepper. Heat a few sprays of low-calorie cooking spray in a large frying pan over a low heat, add the eggs and scramble for 5–6 minutes until cooked through but still soft.

4. Open up the croissants and top with the cheese slices, then the crispy prosciutto, scrambled eggs and chilli jam.

5. Transfer to airtight containers or wrap tightly in tin foil and store in the fridge for up to 3 days.

6. When ready to eat, reheat the croissants in an air fryer at 180°C for 3–4 minutes.

Protein
28.6g

9 780241 693384

Serves: **4**   Prep time: **10 mins**   Cook time: **10 mins**
Cals: **378**   Carbs: **36.5g**   Protein: **11.7g**   Fat: **20.7g**

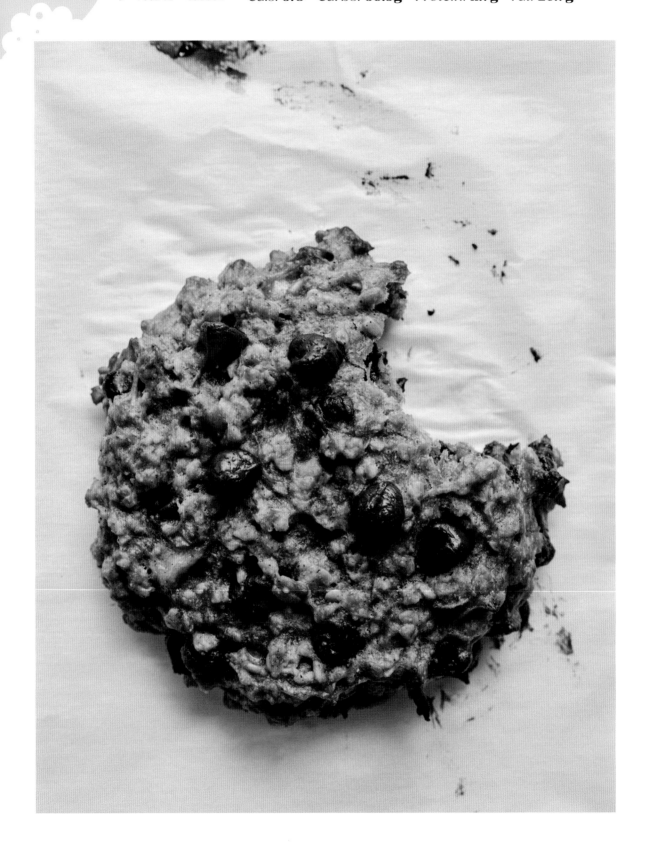

Prep-able Breakfast Cookies

These delicious and healthy five-ingredient oat cookies are naturally sweet and rich thanks to the bananas and peanut butter. Freeze or chill these so you have them to hand to help you stay fuelled throughout the day.

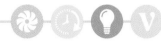

2 ripe bananas
90g jumbo rolled oats
120g smooth peanut butter
½ tsp ground cinnamon
a pinch of salt
50g milk or dark chocolate chips

1. Preheat the oven to 180°C (160°C fan/350°F/Gas 4) and line a baking tray with baking paper.

2. In a bowl, mash the bananas until smooth, then add the oats, peanut butter, cinnamon and salt and mix well. Once combined, fold in the chocolate chips.

3. Divide the mixture into four pieces, then roll into balls and shape into large cookies, about 1–2cm thick and roughly 10cm in diameter. Transfer to the prepared baking tray and bake in the oven for 10–12 minutes until set but still soft. Alternatively, cook in a lined air fryer at 170°C for 6 minutes.

4. Once baked, transfer to an airtight container or wrap in tin foil and store in the fridge for up to 4 days.

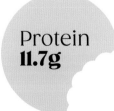

Protein
11.7g

PB & J Protein French Toast

This works perfectly as a make-ahead breakfast, brunch or dessert – or to just enjoy straight away! All you need to do is spread the peanut butter and jam between two luscious brioche slices, soak it in my high-protein French toast mixture and fry or air fry. The brioche will be golden and crispy with a melted, gooey peanut butter and strawberry jam centre – absolutely gorgeous! I really like the fact that this works so well in the air fryer, because it enables you to swap out the butter and save on some calories.

4 eggs
100ml semi-skimmed milk
2 scoops of vanilla protein powder
½ tsp ground cinnamon
½ tsp ground nutmeg
a pinch of salt
3 tbsp smooth or crunchy
  peanut butter
8 slices of brioche
3 tbsp strawberry jam
low-calorie cooking spray (or
  4 small knobs of unsalted butter
  if pan-frying)

To serve
120g Greek yoghurt
4 handfuls of mixed berries
2 tbsp maple syrup

1. In a large bowl, whisk together the eggs, milk, protein powder, cinnamon, nutmeg and salt until there are no lumps of protein powder left.

2. Fold a piece of baking paper two to three times, then place in an air fryer basket (repeat if your air fryer has two drawers).

3. Spread the peanut butter onto half the slices of brioche, then spread the jam onto the other half. Close the sandwiches and dip into the egg mixture.

4. Spray all over with low-calorie cooking spray, then cook in the air fryer at 190°C for 3 minutes on each side. When you flip the French toast, the baking paper will be wet from the uncooked side, so flip the baking paper as well.

   Alternatively, heat a small knob of butter in a non-stick frying pan over a medium heat and fry the French toast for 2–3 minutes on each side until golden and crisp, then repeat with the remaining sandwiches.

5. Allow to cool, then wrap in cling film or transfer to an airtight container and store in the fridge for up to 4 days.

6. Serve with the Greek yoghurt, mixed berries and maple syrup.

Protein
25.1g

Serves: **4**   Prep time: **10 mins**   Cook time: **25 mins**
Cals: **383**   Carbs: **34.1g**   Protein: **25.1g**   Fat: **16.3g**

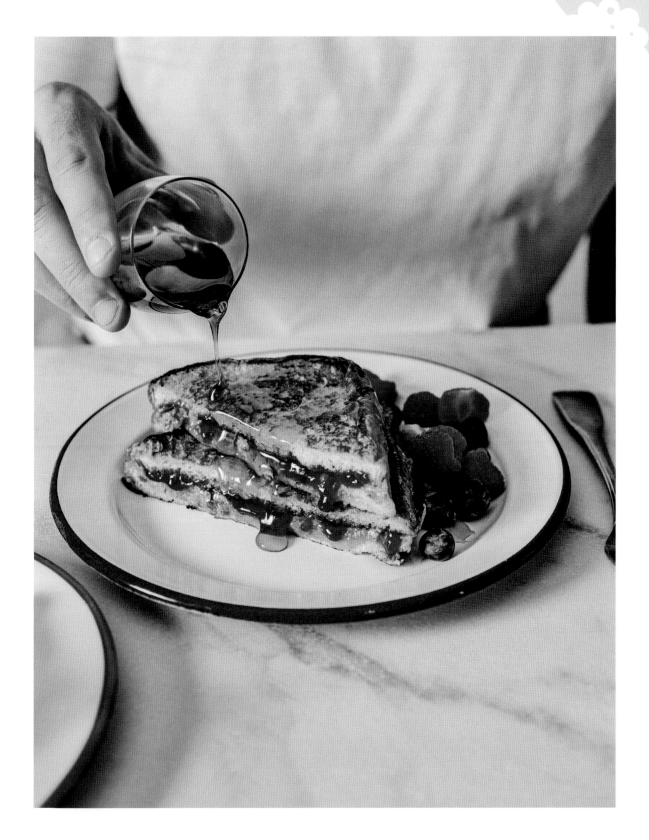

Berry Cheesecake Overnight Oats

This recipe is a little bit like having dessert for breakfast. A high-protein, oaty 'cheesecake', natural mixture is topped with mixed berries. Overnight oats are a staple in my weekly cooking rotation as they take 10 minutes to prepare, are super delicious and are literally designed to be prepped for the week, making them a must-try for you at home.

 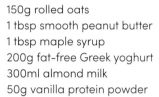

150g rolled oats
1 tbsp smooth peanut butter
1 tbsp maple syrup
200g fat-free Greek yoghurt
300ml almond milk
50g vanilla protein powder

For the topping
400g frozen mixed berries
3 tbsp water

1. First, prepare the berry topping. Put the frozen mixed berries into a saucepan with 3 tablespoons water and cook over a medium heat until the berries are completely broken down, then mash with a potato masher.

2. Meanwhile, mix together the rolled oats, peanut butter, maple syrup, yoghurt, milk and protein powder in a bowl until well combined.

3. Layer the overnight oats into containers or bowls: oat mixture first, then the berry compote. Leave the oats to soak for at least 4 hours or overnight before eating.

4. Store in the fridge for up to 4 days.

Protein
22g

Serves: **4**   Prep time: **5 mins**   Cook time: **5 mins, plus soaking**
Cals: **336**   Carbs: **45.3g**   Protein: **22g**   Fat: **7.6g**

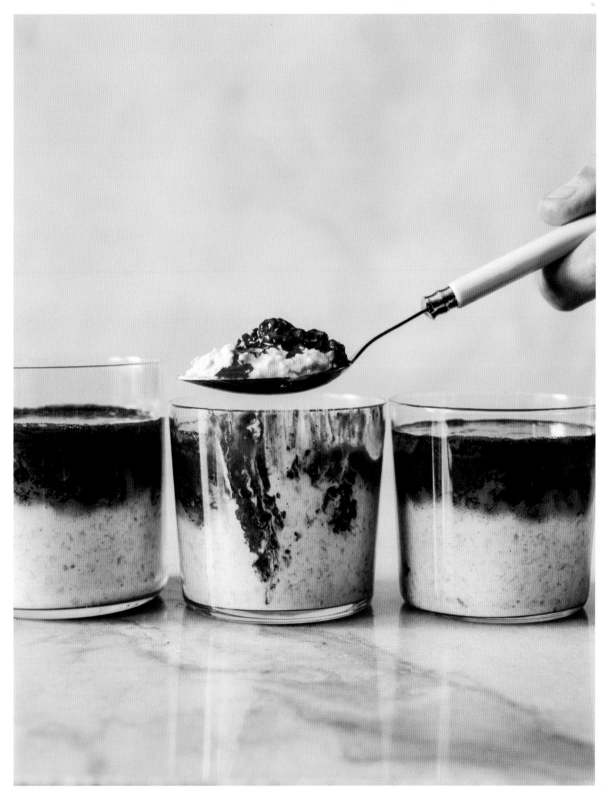

Breakfast Superfood Smoothie

I wanted to create a breakfast smoothie that is perfect for fuelling your day, so that healthy, high-protein living is made easy. These smoothies are packed to the brim with gut-nourishing superfoods.

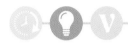

300g frozen mixed berries
75g vanilla protein powder
100g full fat natural or Greek yoghurt
500ml almond milk (or any type of milk)
6 pitted dates
1 tbsp chia seeds
1 tbsp runny honey
2 big handfuls of spinach
50g rolled oats

1. Combine all the ingredients in a blender and blend until smooth.

2. Transfer to four airtight bottles or containers. This will keep in the fridge for up to 4 days.

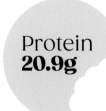

Protein
20.9g

Serves: **4**   Prep time: **2 mins**
Cals: **308**   Carbs: **38.5g**   Protein: **20.9g**   Fat: **8.3g**

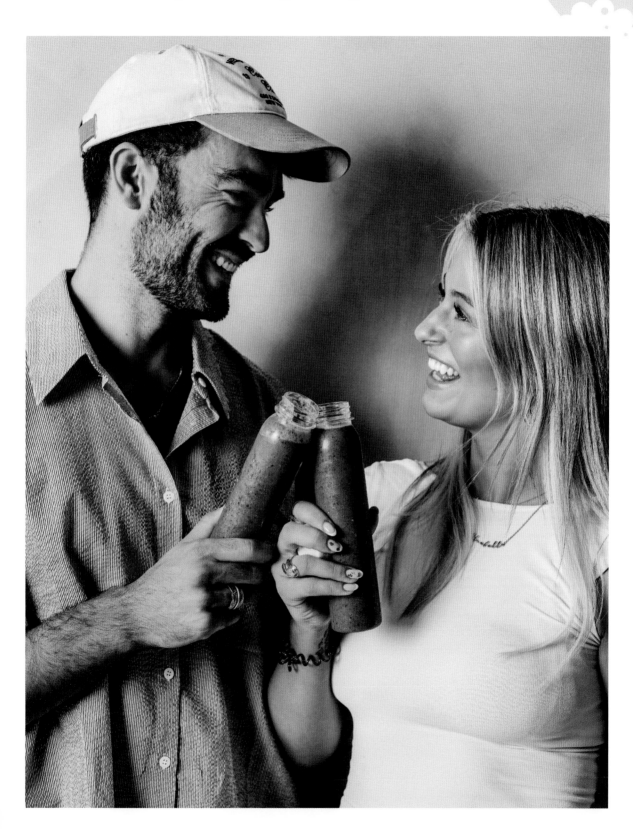

Serves: **4**   Prep time: **5 mins**   Cook time: **45 mins**

Cals: **434**   Carbs: **41.7g**   Protein: **22g**   Fat: **21g**

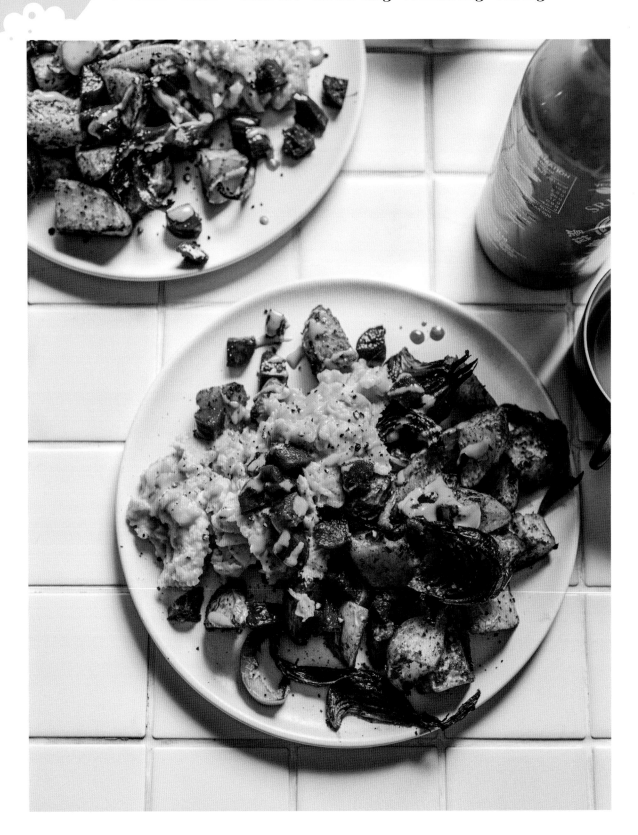

Egg & Chorizo Breakfast Potatoes

Delectable breakfast potatoes, baked with onions, peppers, herbs and spices until golden and crispy, then served with scrambled eggs and crispy chorizo – delicious! This is a straightforward high-protein breakfast that's fit to fuel a champion. Best served hot.

750g Maris Piper potatoes, cut into small cubes
1 tbsp extra virgin olive oil
2 tsp smoked paprika
1 tsp garlic granules
1 tsp onion granules
½ tbsp dried parsley
1 red or green pepper, diced
1 red onion, chopped
8 eggs
2 egg whites
1 tbsp reduced-fat butter spread
60g chorizo, diced
salt and freshly ground
  black pepper
sriracha mayonnaise, to serve
  (optional)

1. Preheat the oven to 200°C (180°C fan/400°F/Gas 6).

2. Put the potatoes into a large bowl and toss with the oil, smoked paprika, garlic granules, onion granules, dried parsley and salt and pepper.

3. Transfer the potatoes to a baking tray, add the pepper and onion and roast in the oven for 30–40 minutes until crispy. Alternatively, cook in an air fryer at 200°C for 25–30 minutes, shaking twice.

4. Meanwhile, whisk together the eggs and egg whites in a bowl. Heat the butter in a large, non-stick frying pan over a low heat and cook the eggs, stirring constantly, until scrambled.

5. Put the chorizo into a small baking dish and bake in the oven or cook in the air fryer for 2–4 minutes until crispy.

6. Divide the breakfast potatoes and eggs between airtight containers, then top with the crispy chorizo and drizzle with the sriracha mayonnaise, if using. This will keep in the fridge for up to 3 days.

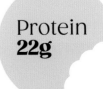

Protein
22g

Chipotle Breakfast Bap

Set yourself up for the day with these super filling and perfectly prep-able breakfast baps. Soft scrambled eggs, streaky bacon and cheese are used to fill a brioche bun, and the icing on the cake is the creamy, spicy and smoky chipotle sauce. Best served hot.

6 eggs
2 egg whites
1 tbsp reduced-fat butter spread
8 rashers of streaky bacon
4 brioche burger buns, toasted
4 American cheese slices
salt and freshly ground
   black pepper

For the chipotle sauce
2 tbsp light mayonnaise
50g reduced-fat crème fraîche
1 tbsp chipotle paste
juice of ½ lime

1. Whisk together the ingredients for the chipotle sauce in a bowl, then set aside.

2. Whisk together the eggs and egg whites in a bowl. Melt the butter in a large, non-stick frying pan over a low heat and cook the eggs, stirring regularly until scrambled. Season to taste.

3. In a separate, non-stick frying pan, cook the bacon over a medium heat until crispy.

4. Build the baps: spread the chipotle sauce on the bottom buns, then top with the eggs, cheese slices and streaky bacon.

5. These will keep in the fridge for up to 4 days.

Protein
24.6g

Serves: **4**   Prep time: **5 mins**   Cook time: **10 mins**
Cals: **448**   Carbs: **27.5g**   Protein: **24.6g**   Fat: **25.9g**

35

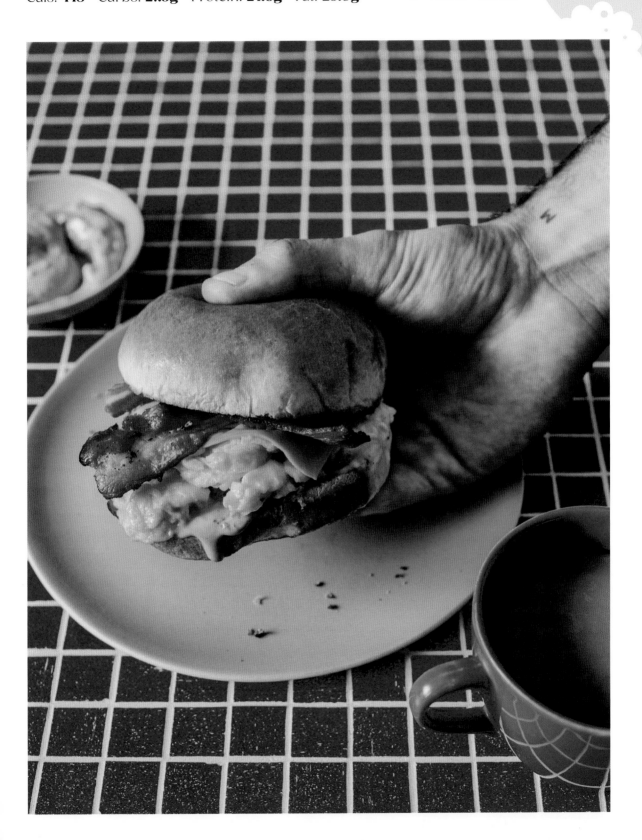

Hot, Hot, Hot Lunches

Spicy Chicken Wraps

Very simple, but absolutely delicious, these are ideal for meal prep, packed lunches or as a quick dinnertime option for the family. They can be served hot or cold.

500g chicken breast, cut into strips
1 tbsp extra virgin olive oil
3–4 cloves of garlic, peeled and
   finely chopped
½ tbsp smoked paprika
1 tsp chilli powder
½ tbsp lemon juice
1 tsp onion granules
½ tbsp dried oregano
salt and freshly ground
   black pepper

For the spicy yoghurt sauce
125g fat-free natural yoghurt
1–2 tbsp sriracha
a handful of fresh coriander or
   parsley, finely chopped

To serve
2 little gem lettuces, chopped
4 tomatoes, diced
½ cucumber, diced
4 tortilla wraps

1. In a large bowl, combine the chicken breast with half the oil and all the remaining ingredients, then season well and mix until combined.

2. In a separate small bowl, combine all the ingredients for the spicy yoghurt.

3. Heat the remaining olive oil in a large, non-stick frying pan over a high heat and add the chicken. Cook for 5–10 minutes, stirring regularly, until the chicken is cooked through and slightly charred.

4. Build your wraps using the lettuce, tomatoes and cucumber, followed by the spicy chicken and sauce. Wrap in cling film or tin foil and store in the fridge for up to 4 days.

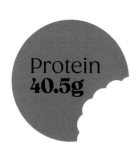

Protein
40.5g

Serves: **4**   Prep time: **10 mins**   Cook time: **10 mins**
Cals: **410**   Carbs: **44.1g**   Protein: **40.5g**   Fat: **9.2g**

39

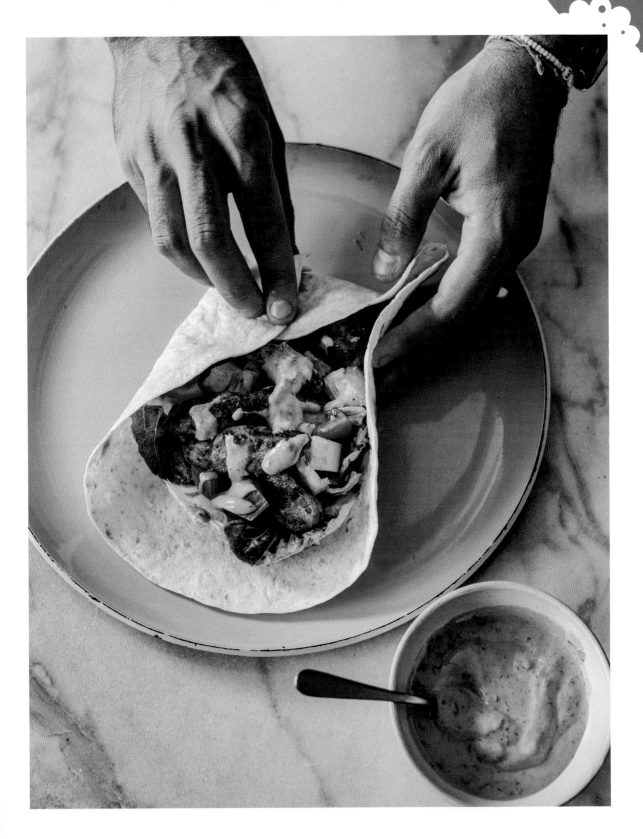

Feta and Orzo Salad
WITH SPICY CHICKPEAS

A light and summery veggie option that is perfect to eat cold. It's also one of the simplest recipes in the whole book. Deli-style, with hot and spicy oven-baked chickpeas coupled up with a refreshing orzo salad and tangy feta.

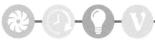

300g orzo
½ tbsp olive oil
juice of ½ lemon
1 red onion, peeled and finely chopped
150g cherry tomatoes, halved
25g fresh basil, chopped
1 tsp dried oregano
½ tsp smoked paprika
120g reduced-fat feta cheese, crumbled or chopped
salt and freshly ground black pepper

For the spicy chickpeas

1 x 400g tin of chickpeas, drained and rinsed
1 tbsp extra virgin olive oil
½ tbsp smoked paprika
1 tsp mild chilli powder
1 tsp garlic granules
1 tsp dried oregano
salt and freshly ground black pepper

1. Preheat oven to 180°C (160°C fan/350°F/Gas 4).

2. Put all the ingredients for the spicy chickpeas into a baking dish, mix well to coat, then bake in the oven for 15 minutes, stirring once. Alternatively, cook in an air fryer at 180°C for 8 minutes.

3. Meanwhile, bring a large saucepan of salted water to the boil and cook the orzo for 6–8 minutes until al dente, then drain and rinse under cold water until completely cooled.

4. Transfer the orzo to a large bowl, then add the oil, lemon juice, red onion, cherry tomatoes, basil, oregano, smoked paprika and 50g of the feta. Season well, then mix until combined.

5. Transfer the orzo salad to airtight containers, then top with spicy chickpeas and remaining feta and store in the fridge for up to 4 days.

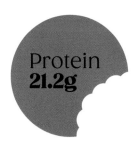

Protein
21.2g

Serves: **4**   Prep time: **10 mins**   Cook time: **15 mins**
Cals: **468**   Carbs: **67.2g**   Protein: **21.2g**   Fat: **11.7g**

41

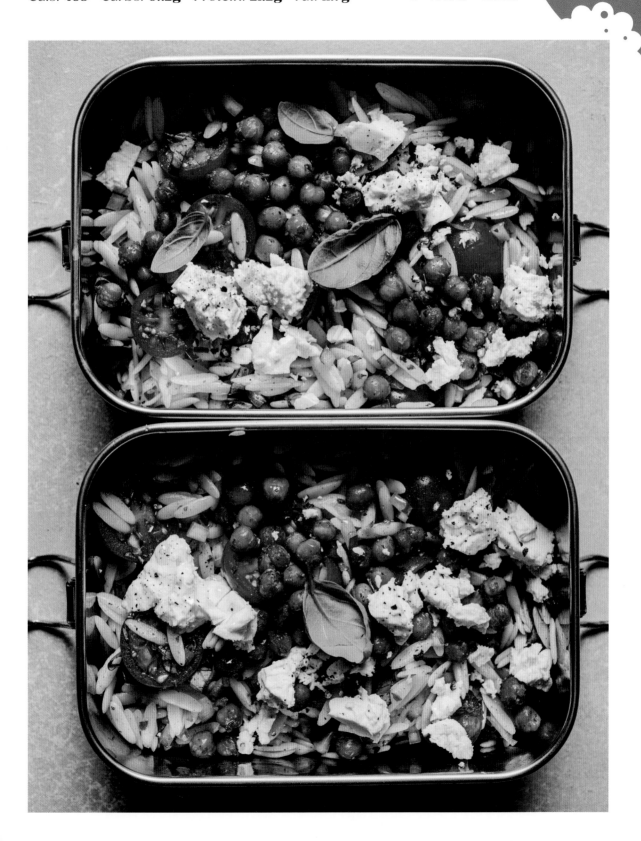

Garlic Butter Chicken Kebabs
WITH LEMON & HERB DIP

Super garlicky and buttery with a citrus kick, these kebabs are amazing. They're low in calories but packed full of flavour and take just over 30 minutes to make. Air fry or bake the kebabs before brushing all over with garlic butter, packing them into your flatbreads or serving with rice and drizzling with a delicious lemon and herb dip.

600g chicken breast, diced
50g fat-free Greek yoghurt
½ tbsp extra virgin olive oil
3–4 cloves of garlic, peeled and finely chopped
juice of 1 lemon
1 tbsp ground cumin
½ tbsp smoked paprika
½ tbsp oregano
½ tsp chilli flakes
salt and freshly ground black pepper

For the lemon and herb dip

75g fat-free Greek yoghurt
juice of ½ lemon
½ tsp ground cumin
½ tbsp dried oregano

For the garlic butter

30g reduced-fat butter spread
1 clove of garlic, peeled and finely chopped

To serve

4 flatbreads or 600g cooked basmati rice
4–6 tomatoes, chopped
1 cucumber, chopped
1 romaine lettuce, chopped

1. Preheat the oven to 180°C (160°C fan/350°F/Gas 4).

2. Combine all the ingredients for the kebabs in a large bowl, season well with salt and pepper and mix until combined, ensuring the chicken is well coated. Divide the chicken among four skewers, then transfer to a large baking tray and bake in the oven for 20–25 minutes. Alternatively, cook in an air fryer at 200°C for 12–15 minutes.

3. Meanwhile, mix together the ingredients for the lemon and herb dip in a bowl, season well with black pepper, then transfer to four sauce pots.

4. Next, make the garlic butter. Put the butter and garlic into a small bowl and microwave on high for 30–45 seconds. Alternatively, melt together in a small pan over a medium heat. Brush the butter over the cooked kebabs.

5. If using flatbreads, then build the flatbreads and wrap tightly in cling film or tin foil. If serving with rice, then transfer the kebabs and rice to airtight containers. Serve with the chopped tomatoes, cucumber and lettuce. This will keep in the fridge for up to 4 days.

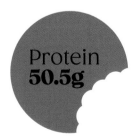

Protein
50.5g

Serves: **4**   Prep time: **10 mins**   Cook time: **25 mins**

With flatbread: Cals: **471**   Carbs: **38.1g**   Protein: **50.5g**   Fat: **11.7g**

With rice: Cals: **443**   Carbs: **46.1g**   Protein: **45.7g**   Fat: **9.4g**

9 780241 693469

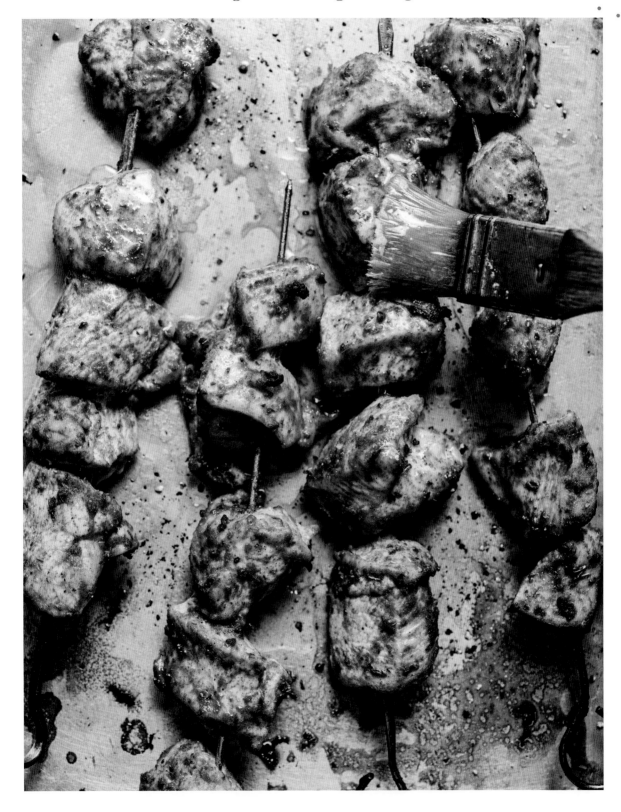

9 780241 693476

Serves: **4**   Prep time: **10 mins**   Cook time: **10 mins**
Cals: **526**   Carbs: **48.9g**   Protein: **32.4g**   Fat: **23.3g**

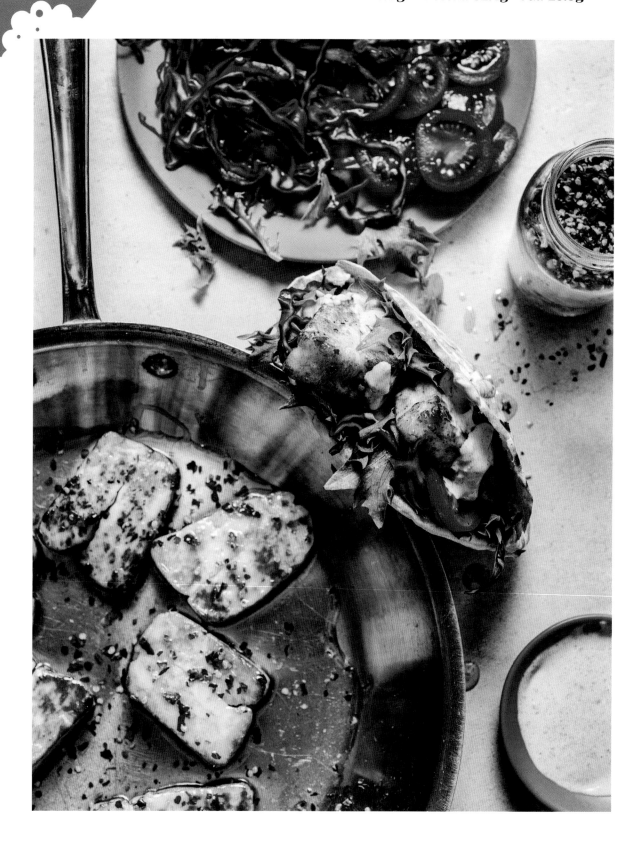

Hot Honey Halloumi Pittas
WITH HARISSA-LIME MAYO

Hot honey and halloumi is a match made in heaven. The blend of sweetness and saltiness just works so well, and pairing it with a super punchy harissa-lime mayo makes for the perfect pitta. These are ready in 10 minutes and are also vegetarian. When ready to eat, you can remove the halloumi and reheat for 45–60 seconds in a microwave or air fryer before adding back to the pitta and eating.

½ small red cabbage, thinly sliced
1 tbsp red wine vinegar
2 x 200g blocks of reduced-fat halloumi, each sliced into 4 pieces
2 tbsp runny honey
1 tsp chilli flakes, or more to taste
1 curly leaf lettuce
4 tomatoes, sliced
4 pitta breads
low-calorie cooking spray

For the harissa-lime mayo
4 tbsp light mayonnaise
1 tbsp harissa paste
juice of 1 lime

1. First, mix together all the ingredients for the harissa-lime mayo in a small bowl and set aside.

2. In a separate large bowl, mix together the red cabbage and vinegar and set aside.

3. Heat a few sprays of low-calorie cooking spray in a large, non-stick frying pan over a high heat and cook the halloumi slices for 2–3 minutes on each side until golden (you may need to do this in batches). Add the honey to the pan along with the chilli flakes and toss until the halloumi slices are coated.

4. Layer the halloumi, lettuce, red cabbage and tomatoes in the pittas, then spread over some harissa-lime mayo. Wrap in cling film or transfer to an airtight container and store in the fridge for up to 4 days.

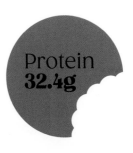

Protein
32.4g

Serves: **4**   Prep time: **10 mins**   Cook time: **15 mins**
Cals: **513**   Carbs: **68g**   Protein: **27.4g**   Fat: **14.8g**

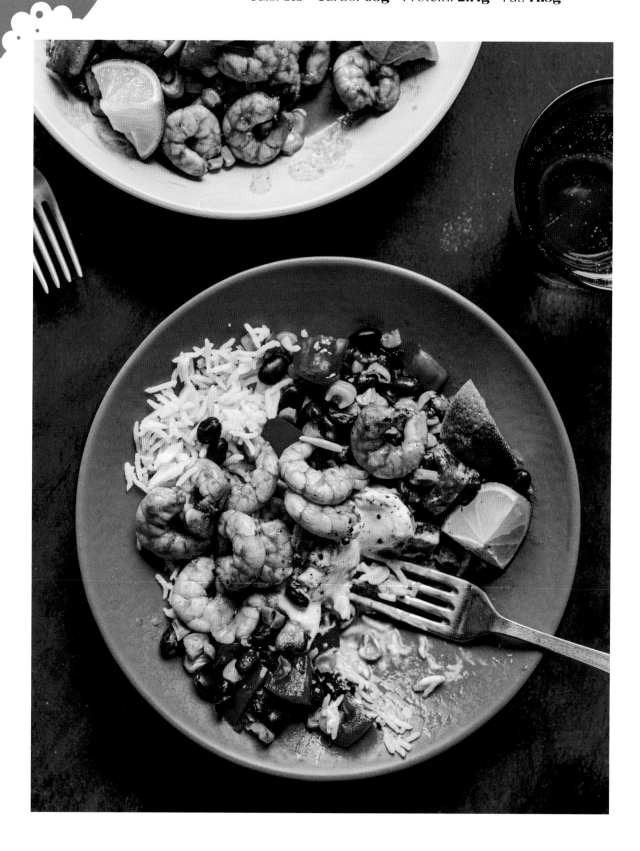

Mexican Prawn Bowl
WITH CORN AND BLACK BEAN SALSA

Juicy king prawns coated in fajita seasoning and lime juice and then air fried, served with the tastiest corn and black bean salsa... My favourite thing about this recipe is the freshness provided by the salsa, which keeps its crunchy texture perfectly even after a few days in the fridge. It also balances so well with the garlicky, salty and spicy prawns. This can be enjoyed hot or cold.

350g raw, unpeeled king prawns
2 cloves of garlic, peeled and thinly sliced
juice of ½ lime
1 tbsp extra virgin olive oil
4 tbsp Fajita Seasoning (see page 158, or use shop-bought)

For the corn and black bean salsa
1 x 340g tin of sweetcorn, drained
1 x 400g tin of black beans, drained
4 tomatoes, chopped
1 fresh jalapeño, deseeded and finely chopped
juice of 1 lime
salt and freshly ground black pepper

For the garlicky soured cream
200g soured cream
1 tsp garlic granules
juice of ½ lime

To serve
4 lime wedges
240g basmati rice

1. First, bring a large saucepan of water to the boil and cook the rice according to packet instructions, then drain.

2. Meanwhile, put the sweetcorn for the salsa into an air fryer basket, season with salt and air fry at 180°C for 10 minutes. Alternatively, fry in a dry frying pan over a medium heat for 5–10 minutes until softened and slightly charred.

3. In a large bowl, combine the prawns, garlic, lime juice, oil and fajita seasoning, then transfer to an air fryer basket and cook for 6–7 minutes, turning once. Alternatively, cook in a non-stick frying pan over a medium heat until pink all over and slightly charred.

4. Combine the sweetcorn with the remaining salsa ingredients in a large bowl, season well and mix until combined.

5. In a separate bowl, combine the garlicky soured cream ingredients, then transfer to sauce pots.

6. Transfer the rice, corn and black bean salsa and king prawns to airtight containers, add the lime wedges and store in the fridge for up to 4 days.

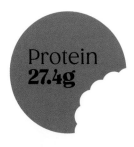

Protein
27.4g

Serves: **4**   Prep time: **5 mins**   Cook time: **25 mins**
Cals: **708**   Carbs: **104.6g**   Protein: **21.9g**   Fat: **19.4g**

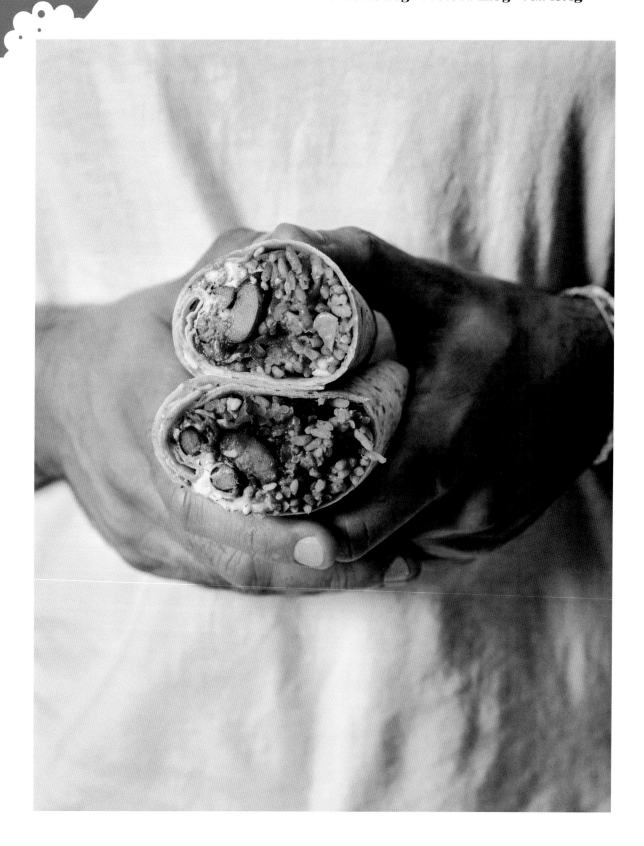

Chipotle Chick'n Burritos

There is nothing better than a burrito for lunch, and this version made with chipotle jackfruit is absolutely divine. I use chipotle chilli paste to instantly achieve that authentic Mexican flavour without needing to soak dried chillies, and I serve the jackfruit with a zesty coconut yoghurt sauce to compliment the spice. What's even better is that it is all 100 per cent plant-based.

1 tbsp olive or groundnut oil
1 onion, thinly sliced
2 cloves of garlic, peeled and
  finely chopped
1 x 400g tins of jackfruit
1 x 400g tin of kidney beans,
  drained and rinsed
2 tbsp chipotle paste
1 tsp ground cumin
1 tsp smoked paprika
1 tsp mild chilli powder
½ tsp ground cinnamon
½ tsp ground coriander
1 x 400g tin of chopped tomatoes
200ml vegetable stock

For the zesty coconut yoghurt sauce

200g coconut yoghurt
a handful of fresh coriander,
  finely chopped
juice of ½ lime

To serve

4 tortilla wraps
2 x 250g packets of Mexican
  microwave rice
1 x 400g tin of black beans,
  drained and rinsed
50g plant-based cheese, grated
a handful of fresh coriander,
  chopped

1. Heat the oil in a non-stick frying pan over a low heat and cook the onion for 5 minutes, then add the garlic and cook for a further 1–2 minutes until soft.

2. Meanwhile, drain the jackfruit and transfer to a large bowl. Use your hands to pull it apart into thin strands until completely shredded.

3. Add the shredded jackfruit, kidney beans, chipotle paste, cumin, smoked paprika, chilli powder, cinnamon and coriander to the pan and stir everything together. Cook for 2 minutes, then add the chopped tomatoes and vegetable stock, bring to a rapid simmer and allow to reduce for 10–15 minutes until thickened.

4. Meanwhile, mix together the coconut yoghurt, coriander and lime juice in a bowl to create your zesty yoghurt sauce.

5. Build your burritos using the tortilla wraps, Mexican rice, chipotle jackfruit filling, black beans, plant-based cheese, coriander and yoghurt sauce. Tightly wrap in tin foil and store in the fridge for 3–4 days.

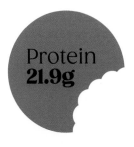

Protein
21.9g

Creamy Tuscan Butter Beans

Butter beans braised in a rich and creamy Tuscan sauce make a quick
and easy vegetarian option that is full of bold and comforting flavours.

1 tbsp extra virgin olive oil

2 shallots, peeled and finely
chopped

2 cloves of garlic, peeled
and crushed

1 sweet Romano pepper,
finely chopped

1 tbsp tomato purée

2 x 400g tins of butter beans,
drained

300ml vegetable stock

½ tbsp dried oregano

a pinch of chilli flakes

75g reduced-fat crème fraîche

1 tbsp light cream cheese

1 tsp smoked paprika

300g cherry tomatoes

a handful of spinach

salt and freshly ground
black pepper

4 slices of toasted sourdough
bread, to serve

1. Heat the olive oil in a large saucepan over a medium heat and
fry the shallots, garlic and Romano pepper for 5 minutes until
softened. Increase the heat to high, add the tomato purée, stir
well and fry for 2 minutes. Add the butter beans, vegetable stock,
oregano and chilli flakes, then bring to a low simmer and allow to
reduce for 10 minutes.

2. Once reduced, turn down the heat to low and add the crème
fraîche, cream cheese, smoked paprika and tomatoes. Stir
to combine, then simmer the sauce for 5–10 minutes until the
tomatoes are just about bursting but still whole. Stir in the spinach
and cook for 2–3 minutes until wilted, then season with salt and
pepper and remove from the heat.

3. Transfer to airtight containers and store in the fridge for 3–4 days.
Serve with the toasted sourdough.

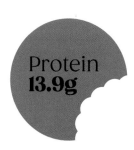

Protein
13.9g

Serves: **4**   Prep time: **5 mins**   Cook time: **30 mins**

Cals: **331**   Carbs: **46.3g**   Protein: **13.9g**   Fat: **8.6g**

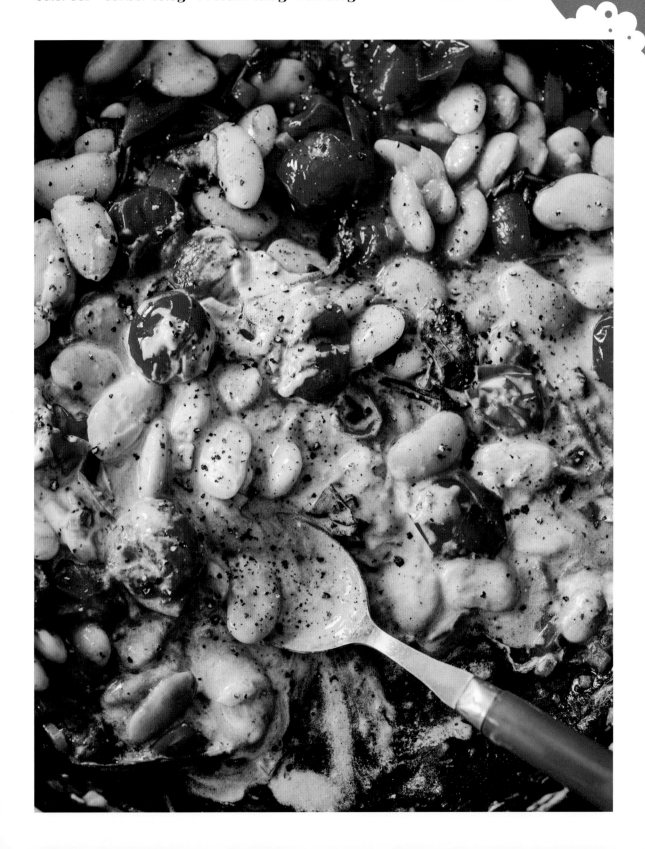

Serves: **4** Prep time: **5 mins** Cook time: **25 mins**
Cals: **576** Carbs: **68.7g** Protein: **29.1g** Fat: **22g**

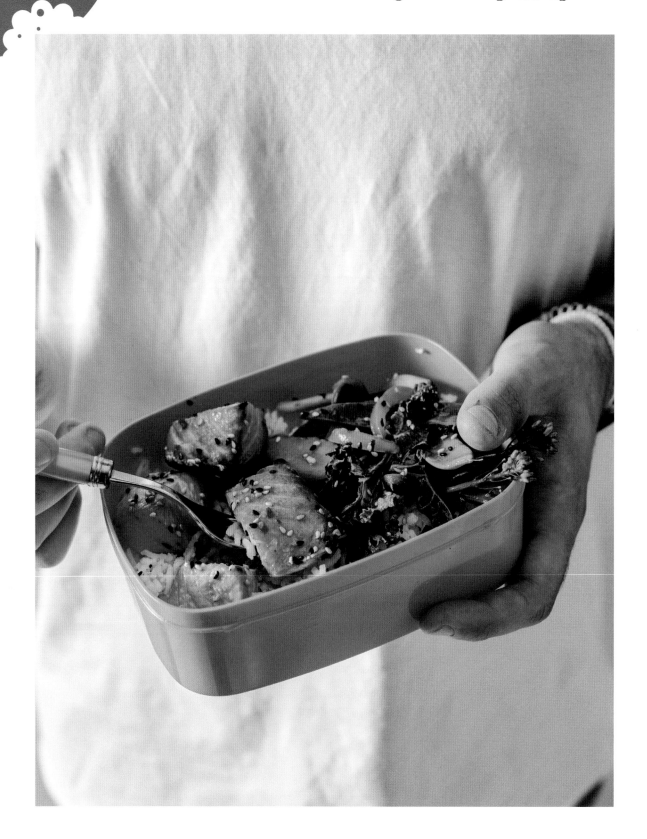

Hot Honey Garlic Salmon Bites
WITH STIR-FRIED VEG

I love these garlicky salmon bites, air fried until crispy, then tossed in a moreish, sweet and spicy hot honey sauce. Here, I've served them with fluffy basmati rice and crunchy stir-fried vegetables. This is a balanced and super tasty meal prep option with loads of health benefits provided by the salmon.

4 tbsp runny honey
2 tbsp light soy sauce
1 clove of garlic, peeled
  and crushed
1 tsp chilli flakes
420g salmon fillet, cut into
  bite-sized pieces

To serve
240g basmati rice
½ tbsp groundnut oil
1 x 250g pack of stir-fry vegetables
3 spring onions, chopped
1 tbsp white sesame seeds
1 tbsp black sesame seeds

1. First, bring a large saucepan of water to the boil and cook the rice according to the packet instructions, then drain.

2. If not using an air fryer, preheat the oven to 180°C (160°C fan/350°F/Gas 4) and line a baking tray with baking paper.

3. Whisk together the honey, soy sauce, garlic and chilli flakes in a bowl.

4. Put the salmon pieces into a large bowl with half the sauce and stir to coat. Line an air fryer basket (or baskets) with baking paper and cook in two batches at 190°C for 8 minutes, flipping once. Alternatively, transfer the salmon bites to the prepared baking tray and bake in the oven for 12–15 minutes until crispy.

5. Meanwhile, mix 2 tablespoons water with the remaining sauce in a frying pan over a low heat and simmer gently for 3 minutes, stirring constantly, then transfer to sauce pots.

6. In the same pan, heat the groundnut oil over a medium heat and stir-fry the mixed vegetables for 3–4 minutes, then remove from heat.

7. Transfer the rice, salmon bites and vegetables to airtight containers and garnish with the spring onions and sesame seeds. Store in the fridge for up to 3 days.

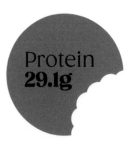

Protein
29.1g

Halloumi & Sweet Chilli Jam Flatbreads

These halloumi kebabs are dusted with smoked paprika and air fried until golden and crisp before being coated in an amazing three-ingredient sticky sweet chilli jam. Wrap them up into a flatbread with my simple yoghurt-based garlic and lime dip to make the perfect quick and easy high-protein veggie meal prep.

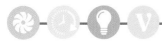

2 x 200g blocks of reduced-fat halloumi cheese, cut into 2–3cm cubes
2 peppers, chopped
1 tsp smoked paprika
150g fat-free Greek yoghurt
1 tsp garlic granules
juice of 1 lime
4 flatbreads
1 small romaine lettuce, leaves separated
2 spring onions, finely chopped
low-calorie cooking spray

For the sweet chilli jam
2 tbsp reduced-sugar sweet chilli sauce
2 tbsp chilli jam
juice of 1 lime

1. Thread the halloumi and peppers onto skewers, then sprinkle with the smoked paprika and spray all over with low-calorie cooking spray. Cook in an air fryer at 200°C for 8 minutes. Alternatively, heat ½ tablespoon of oil in a non-stick pan and fry the halloumi skewers for 2 minutes on each side, until golden and crispy.

2. Meanwhile, mix together the ingredients for the sweet chilli jam in a small bowl.

3. In a separate bowl, mix together the yoghurt, garlic granules and lime juice.

4. Remove the skewers from the air fryer and brush the skewers with most of the chilli jam, then return to the air fryer for a further 2 minutes.

5. Spread the flatbreads with the garlic yoghurt, then top with the lettuce leaves, halloumi skewers, spring onions and reserved chilli jam. These will keep in the fridge for up to 4 days.

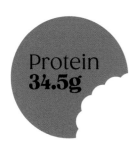

Protein
34.5g

9 780241 693520

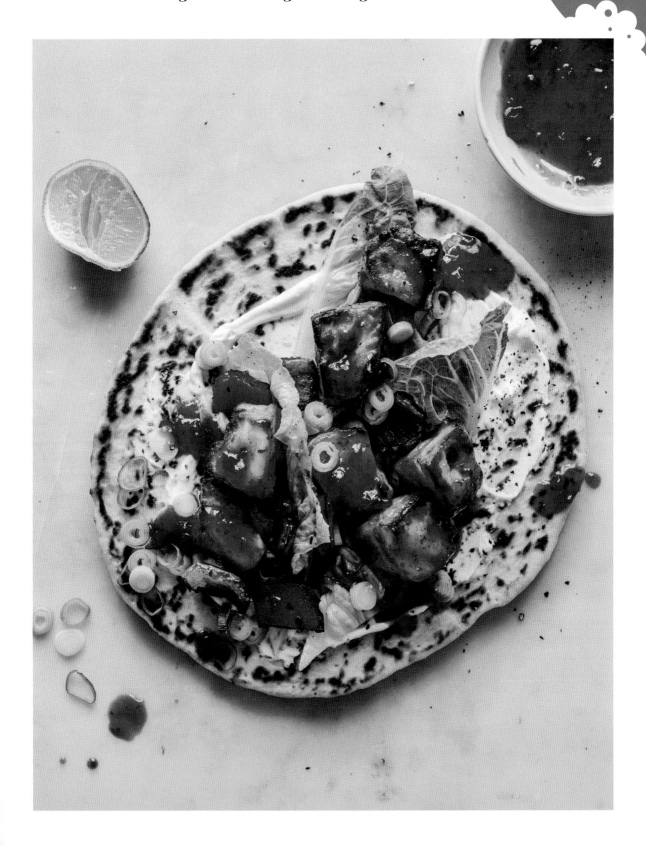

Peri-peri Butterfly Chicken
WITH SQUASH, GRAINS & FETA SALAD

This one is definitely inspired by Nando's. I've combined a light and super-fresh grain salad with the perfect balance of sweet butternut squash and salty, tangy feta, all topped with a grilled, spicy peri-peri butterfly chicken breast. This is a delicious and nutritionally complete meal that keeps perfectly as meal prep.

2 large chicken breasts
3–4 tbsp peri-peri sauce
1 tbsp extra virgin olive oil

For the squash, grains and feta salad

180g mixed grains, such as bulgur wheat and white and red quinoa, rinsed
1 small butternut squash, peeled and cut into 2cm chunks
1 tbsp extra virgin olive oil
1 tsp ground cumin
1 tsp smoked paprika
100g reduced-fat feta cheese, crumbled
40g pomegranate seeds
a small bunch of fresh parsley, chopped
juice of 1 lemon
salt and freshly ground black pepper

1. Preheat the oven to 200°C (180°C fan/400°F/Gas 6) and line a baking tray with baking paper.

2. Bring a large saucepan of water to the boil and cook the grains for 12 minutes, or until soft and tender, then drain into a sieve and leave to steam.

3. Meanwhile, put the squash onto the prepared baking tray, drizzle with half the oil and season with salt and pepper. Bake for 12–15 minutes, turning once, until soft. Alternatively cook in an air fryer at 180°C for 8-10 minutes, or until soft.

4. Next, make the chicken. Lay the chicken breasts flat on a board and butterfly them by slicing each one down the side to create four thinner breasts. Transfer to large bowl and add 2 tablespoons of the peri-peri sauce, then stir to coat. Heat the oil in a cast-iron griddle pan or frying pan over a medium heat and cook the chicken for 4–5 minutes on each side until cooked through and charred. Alternatively, cook in an air fryer at 190°C for 12–15 minutes, or until cooked through. Once cooked, brush with remaining peri-peri sauce.

5. Put the cooked grains into a large bowl with the butternut squash and all the remaining salad ingredients and gently toss to combine, being careful not to squash the butternut squash.

6. Transfer the salad and chicken to airtight containers and store in the fridge for up 4 days.

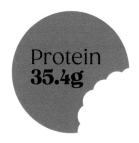

Protein
35.4g

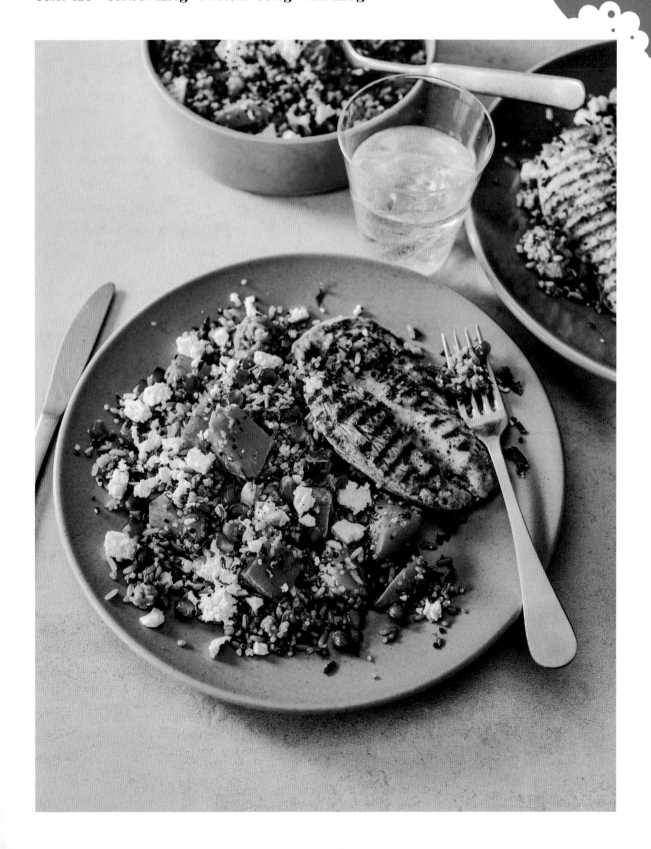

Air-fryer Gyros
WITH CHUNKY TZATZIKI

Juicy and herby chicken thighs, wrapped up in a flatbread with chips and a refreshing and cool chunky tzataziki – heaven! Everybody loves a gyros, and it was actually the first thing I ate the morning after my wedding on the Greek island of Paxos. I was feeling slightly worse for wear, as I'm sure you can imagine, but the delicious gyros sorted me out! I dare say my gyros are a tad healthier than the one I had that morning, but they still pack in a load of flavour. These work amazingly air fried, and you can chuck the chicken and chips in the air fryer (or oven) at the same time, meaning everything can be ready in 25 minutes. I've kept the tzatziki chunky because I like the crunchy texture it provides as well as saving time, not grating the cucumber.

500g boneless, skinless chicken thighs (can be swapped for chicken breast)
½ tbsp extra virgin olive oil
½ tbsp red wine vinegar
juice of ½ lemon
3 cloves of garlic, peeled and finely grated
1 tsp ground cumin
1 tsp smoked paprika
1 tsp dried oregano
1 tsp salt
freshly ground black pepper

For the tzatziki

250g fat-free yoghurt
1 clove of garlic, peeled and grated
a handful of fresh mint leaves, finely chopped
1 small cucumber, chopped
juice of ½ lemon
freshly ground black pepper

To serve

100g frozen French fries
4 flatbreads
½ small red cabbage, thinly sliced
150g cherry tomatoes, halved

1. If not using an air fryer, preheat the oven to 180°C (160°C fan/350°F/Gas 4).

2. Put the chicken thighs into a large bowl with the oil, vinegar, lemon juice, garlic, cumin, smoked paprika, oregano, salt and plenty of black pepper and mix well until the chicken is coated. Transfer to an air fryer and cook at 190°C for 15 minutes. Alternatively, transfer the chicken thighs to a baking dish or loaf tin and cook in the oven for 25 minutes until cooked through.

3. In a separate air fryer basket (or immediately after the chicken is cooked), cook the French fries according to the packet instructions. If using one place in the oven at 180°C (160°C fan/350°F/Gas 4) for 30 minutes.

4. Meanwhile, mix together all the ingredients for the tzatziki in a bowl, then transfer to sauce pots.

5. Build the gyros wraps using the flatbreads, chicken, red cabbage and tomatoes, then wrap tightly in tin foil and store in the fridge for 3–4 days. If eating the gyros straight away add the French fries, but if you're meal prepping leave them out and add them fresh on the day.

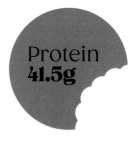

Protein
41.5g

Serves: **4**   Prep time: **5 mins**   Cook time: **25 mins**
Cals: **596**   Carbs: **54.3g**   Protein: **41.5g**   Fat: **21.4g**

59

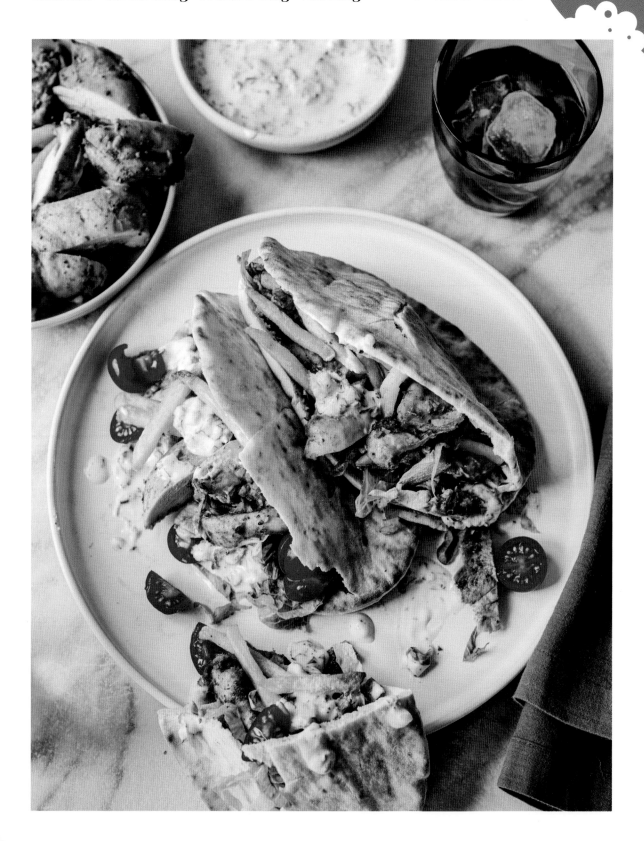

Sandwiches
& Salads

Egg Mayo & Prosciutto Sarnie

This is my lighter version of an egg mayo sandwich, but of course no flavour has been sacrificed. I've swapped out mayonnaise for fat-free yoghurt and added crispy prosciutto instead of bacon. Prosciutto is surprisingly light in calories but packs so much flavour.

8 eggs
6 slices of prosciutto
200g fat-free Greek yoghurt
½ tbsp Dijon mustard
1 tbsp white wine vinegar
20g fresh chives, chopped
a pinch of chilli flakes
8 slices of thick white bread
a couple of handfuls of watercress
low-calorie cooking spray
salt and freshly ground
   black pepper

1. Bring a large saucepan of water to the boil and cook the eggs for 10 minutes, then transfer to a bowl of cold water and leave to cool for 5 minutes.

2. Meanwhile, cook the prosciutto slices in an air fryer at 200°C for 5–7 minutes until very crisp, then remove and chop into fine pieces. Alternatively, heat a few sprays of low-calorie cooking spray in a non-stick pan and cook for 5–7 minutes until crispy.

3. Once cooled, peel the eggs and separate the yolks from the whites. Transfer the egg yolks to a large bowl and mash with the yoghurt, mustard and vinegar. Chop the egg whites and add to the bowl along with the chives, chilli flakes and salt and pepper, then stir to combine.

4. Lightly toast the bread, then top half the slices with the watercress, egg mayo mixture and the crispy prosciutto. Place the other slices on top and cut each sandwich in half, then tightly wrap in tin foil.

5. Store in the fridge for up to 3 days.

Protein
30.7g

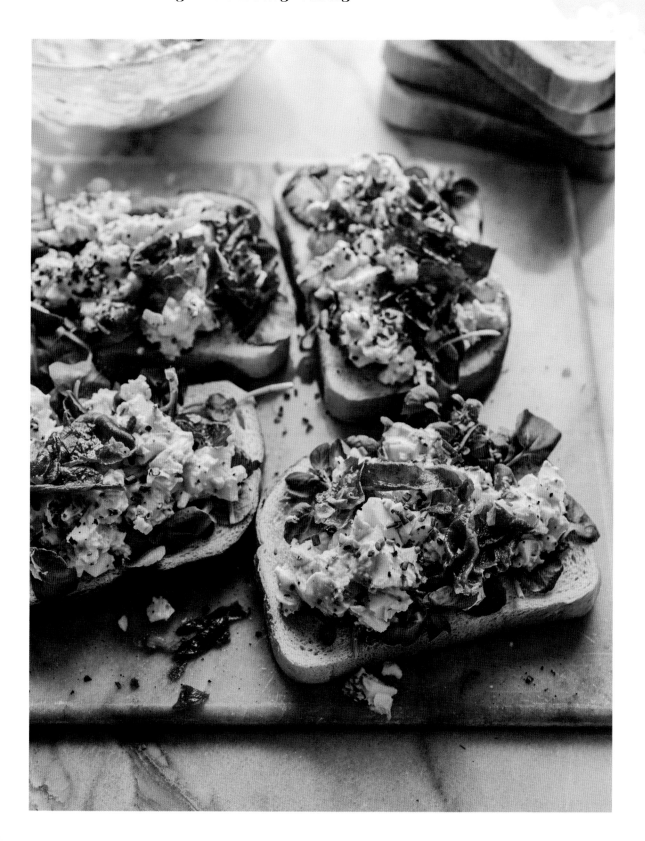

Serves: **4**   Prep time: **10 mins**   Cook time: **40 mins**
Cals: **494**   Carbs: **50.1g**   Protein: **29.5g**   Fat: **20.5g**

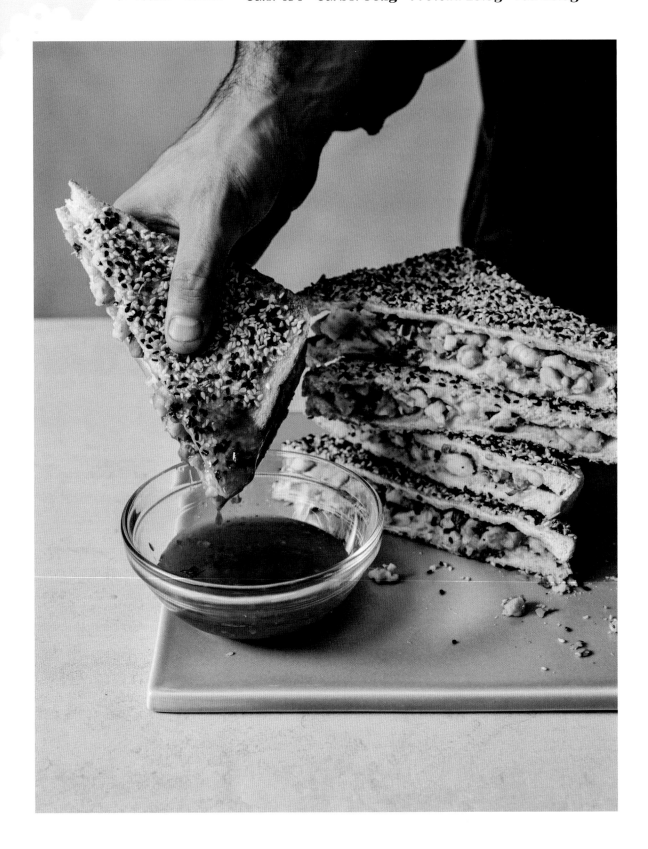

Air-fryer Prawn Toast Toasties

If you're a fan of prawn toast, then you need to try these prawn toast toasties for lunch! The filling is super easy and takes minutes to mix together, then you pack it in between two slices of bread, dip in egg, coat in sesame seeds and air fry. The vibrant and punchy flavour combination of the spring onions, ginger, garlic and chilli is delicious and the sesame seeds create a moreish crunchy exterior.

300g peeled, raw prawns, finely chopped

a small bunch of fresh coriander, finely chopped

6 spring onions, finely chopped

10g fresh ginger, peeled and finely grated to make a paste

1 clove of garlic, peeled and finely grated to make a paste

1 tbsp light soy sauce

a pinch of chilli flakes

3 egg yolks

8 slices of thick white bread

4 tbsp black sesame seeds

4 tbsp white sesame seeds

3 egg whites

low-calorie cooking spray

sweet chilli sauce, to serve

1. Put the prawns, coriander, spring onions, ginger, garlic, soy sauce, chilli flakes and egg yolks into a large bowl and mix until combined.

2. Lay half the slices of bread out on a surface and spread with the prawn mixture, then top with the remaining slices.

3. In a small bowl, mix together the black and white sesame seeds.

4. Lightly whisk the egg whites in a bowl until combined, then dip each sandwich in the egg whites before sprinkling all over with the mixed sesame seeds. Spray all over with low-calorie cooking spray and cook in an air fryer at 180°C for 4–5 minutes on each side until golden and crispy. Alternatively, heat a little cooking spray or oil in a frying pan and fry for 4–5 minutes on each side.

5. Depending on how big your air fryer or pan is you'll have to cook your toasties in batches, which is why I've left lots of room in the cooking time.

6. Wrap tightly in cling film or tin foil and store in the fridge for up to 4 days.

Protein
29.5g

Chicken Souvlaki
WITH GREEK SALAD

This is my take on super garlicky, zingy chicken souvlaki combined with crisp, fresh vegetables and all tied together by a punchy feta dressing. This recipe was inspired by the many trips that my wife, Megan, and I have taken to the Greek island of Paxos, where we tied the knot! The feta dressing is something you might not usually do for a Greek salad, but it takes it to the next level. I really wanted to ensure this meal stays fresh for as long as possible, and I've achieved this by draining some of the tomato juice before making the salad. Storing the feta dressing in sauce pots and mixing it in just before serving also helps to keep things crunchy and full of flavour. The chicken skewers can be served either hot or cold.

100g 5% fat Greek yoghurt
½ tbsp extra virgin olive oil
juice of 1 lemon
5 cloves of garlic, peeled and crushed
1½ tbsp dried oregano
1 tsp salt
freshly ground black pepper
450g chicken breast, diced
low-calorie cooking spray, if needed
2 pitta breads, halved, to serve

For the feta dressing
2 tbsp extra virgin olive oil
1 tbsp red wine vinegar
juice of ½ lemon
½ tbsp dried oregano
50g reduced-fat feta cheese

For the Greek salad
6–8 vine-ripened tomatoes, diced
a pinch of flaky sea salt
2 green peppers, chopped
1 large cucumber, chopped
½ red onion, thinly sliced
50g pitted kalamata olives, chopped
100g reduced-fat feta cheese, crumbled

1. First, put the tomatoes for the salad into a colander with the salt and set aside to allow the tomato juice to drain while you prepare everything else.

2. Combine the yoghurt, oil, lemon juice, garlic, oregano, salt and plenty of black pepper in a large bowl and mix well, then add the chicken and mix again.

3. Thread the chicken onto skewers, then transfer to an air fryer basket and cook at 200°C for 12–15 minutes until cooked through and charred. Alternatively, heat a few sprays of low-calorie cooking spray in a non-stick frying pan over a medium heat and cook the chicken for 10 minutes, flipping once or twice.

4. Meanwhile, make the feta dressing. Combine the oil, vinegar, lemon juice and oregano in a bowl, then add the feta and mash using the back of a fork to create a thick dressing. Transfer to sauce pots.

5. In a large bowl, mix together all the ingredients for the salad, then divide into airtight containers and crumble the feta over the top. Add the chicken and pittas and store in the fridge for up to 4 days.

Protein
42.3g

Serves: **4**   Prep time: **15 mins**   Cook time: **15 mins**

Cals: **511**   Carbs: **23.7g**   Protein: **42.3g**   Fat: **28g**

9 780241 693575

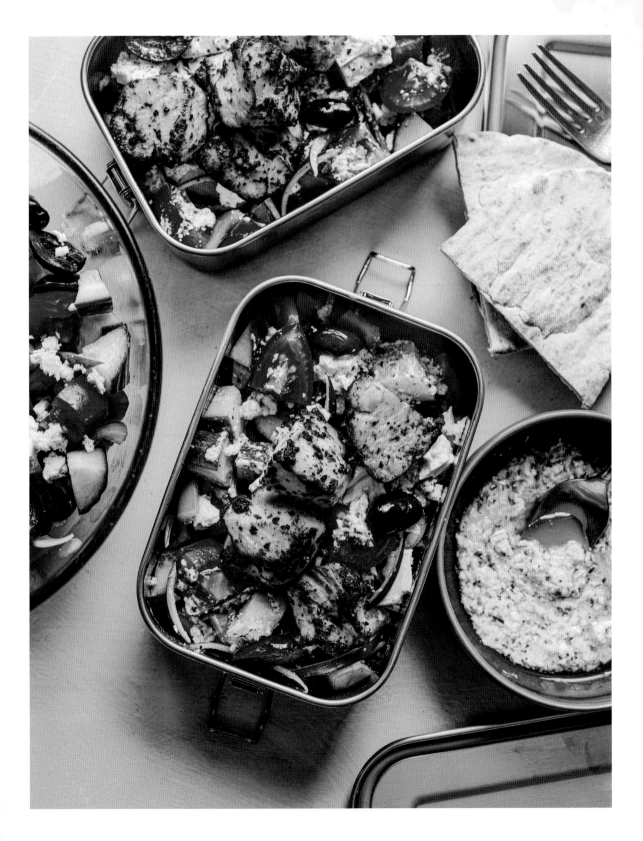

9 780241 693582

Serves: **4**   Prep time: **10 mins**   Cook time: **10 mins**
Cals: **465**   Carbs: **36.9g**   Protein: **15.7g**   Fat: **27.7g**

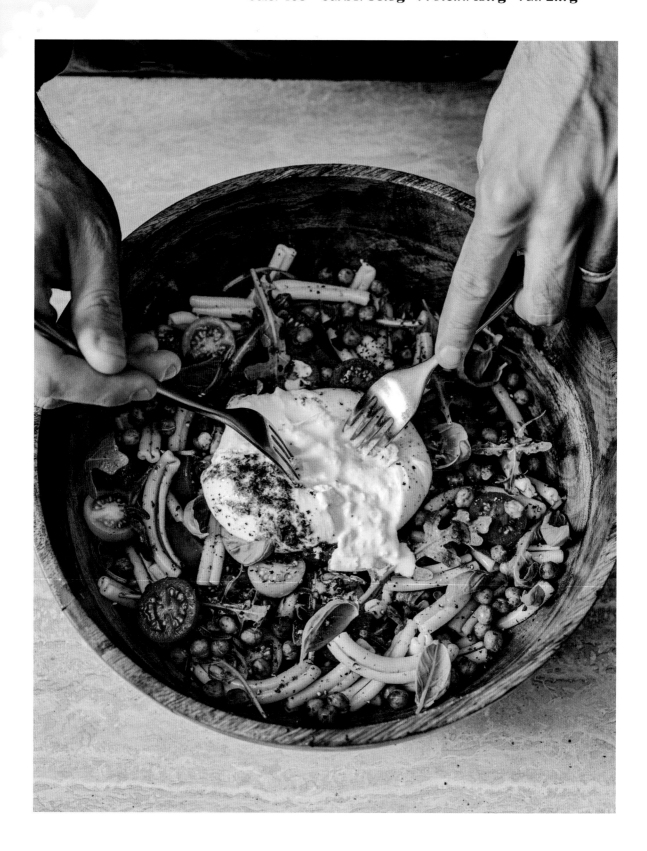

Burrata Pasta Salad
WITH CRISPY CHICKPEAS & BASIL DRESSING

This is a low-calorie and nutritionally complete pasta salad that is perfect for summer. The creaminess of the burrata with the crunchy, crispy texture of the chickpeas and the light and delicate basil dressing makes for a combination that is out of this world.

250g casarecce, or similar pasta
1 x 400g tin of chickpeas, drained
1 tsp smoked paprika
1 tsp garlic granules
½ tbsp extra virgin olive oil
300g mixed cherry tomatoes, halved
2 peppers (any colour), chopped
60g rocket
1 burrata, torn
small bunch of fresh basil, whole leaves
salt and freshly ground black pepper

For the basil dressing
1½ tbsp extra virgin olive oil
10g fresh basil
1 clove of garlic, peeled and crushed
juice of 1 lemon
a pinch of salt

1. Preheat the oven to 200°C (180°C fan/400°F/Gas 6) and line a baking tray with baking paper.

2. Bring a large saucepan of salted water to the boil and cook the pasta until al dente, then drain and rinse under cold water until completely cool.

3. Meanwhile, pat the chickpeas dry with kitchen paper, then transfer to a bowl and add the smoked paprika, garlic granules and plenty of salt and pepper and ½ tablespoon of olive oil. Toss to coat, then transfer to the prepared baking tray and bake in the oven for 8–10 minutes until crispy. Alternatively, cook in an air fryer at 200°C for 6–8 minutes.

4. Meanwhile, combine all the ingredients for the basil dressing in a jug or bowl and use a hand-held blender to blend until fully combined.

5. Put the pasta, chickpeas, tomatoes, peppers and rocket into a large bowl, drizzle over the basil dressing and mix well. Add the burrata and fresh basil, then mix again.

6. Transfer to airtight containers and store in the fridge for up to 4 days.

Protein
15.7g

9 780241 693599

Serves: **4**   Prep time: **5 mins**   Cook time: **10 mins**
Cals: **557**   Carbs: **70.2g**   Protein: **30.3g**   Fat: **17.2g**

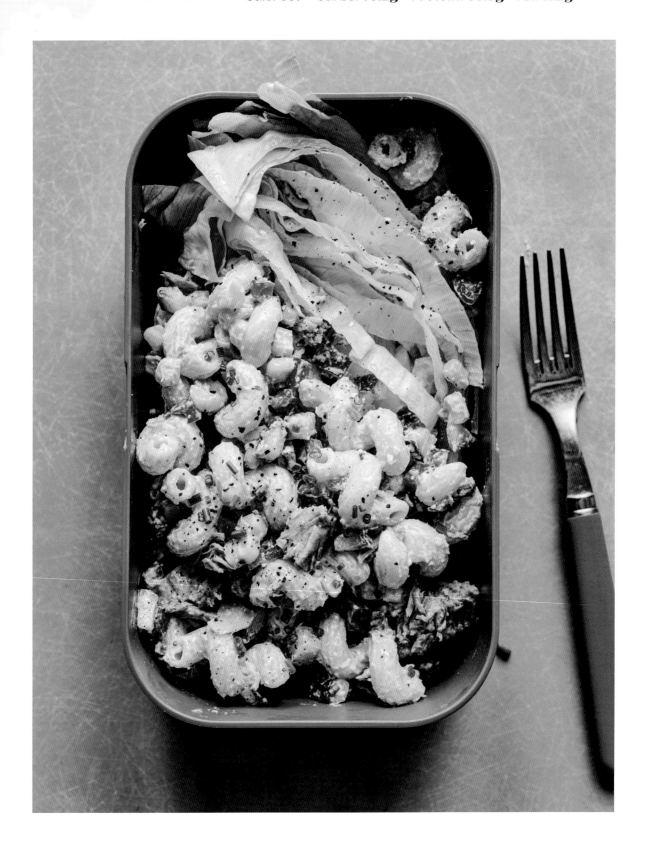

My Perfect Tuna Pasta Salad

This is a recipe I came up with on a lazy Sunday afternoon when I fancied something quick and easy. Tuna pasta salad is a well-known classic, but I think mine really benefits from the addition of the rich and salty Parmesan and crème fraîche for creaminess. This is light and fresh, perfect for fuelling your day – and it's ready in as long as it takes for the pasta to cook! Best served cold.

300g spirali, or similar pasta
1 tbsp extra virgin olive oil
4 tbsp light mayonnaise
4 tbsp reduced-fat crème fraîche
juice of 1 lemon
½ tbsp Dijon mustard
3 x 112g tins of tuna, drained
1 cucumber, deseeded
  and chopped
1 red pepper, chopped
1 x 340g tin of sweetcorn, drained
a handful of fresh chives, chopped
½ iceberg lettuce, thinly sliced
½ tbsp dried parsley
30g Parmesan, grated
salt and freshly ground
  black pepper

1. Bring a large saucepan of salted water to the boil and cook the pasta until al dente, then drain and rinse under cold water until completely cool.

2. Meanwhile, in a large bowl, mix together the oil, mayonnaise, crème fraîche, lemon juice and mustard, then add all the remaining ingredients. Mix well and season to taste.

3. Transfer to airtight containers and store in the fridge for up to 4 days.

Protein
30.3g

Harissa & Tahini Jar Salads

Jar salads are an awesome meal-prep food hack. They're quick, perfect for storing, easy to experiment with and result in a fresh and super delicious salad for you to enjoy on your lunch break. Just pack your jars with a dressing, plant-based protein option such as chickpeas or lentils, carbohydrates such as pasta or couscous, then add your salad. I've used a mixture of harissa and tahini for the dressing to provide a lovely smoky and nutty flavour. The best part is that the protein options soak up all those delicious flavours as they're left to marinate in the dressing.

1 cucumber, chopped
1 red onion, finely chopped
300g cherry tomatoes, halved
1 romaine lettuce, chopped

Carb options (pick one):
200g farfalle, or similar pasta
200g couscous

Protein options (pick one):
1 x 400g tin of kidney beans
1 x 400g tin of black beans
1 x 400g tin of lentils
1 x 400g tin of chickpeas

For the dressing (per jar):
½ tbsp extra virgin olive oil
½ tbsp harissa paste
1 tbsp tahini
1 tbsp or a squeeze of lemon juice
1 tsp runny honey or agave syrup
a pinch of sea salt
1 tbsp water

1. If using pasta, bring a large saucepan of salted water to the boil and cook the pasta until al dente, then drain and rinse under cold water. If using couscous, combine the couscous with 200ml boiling water in a large bowl, cover for 6 minutes, then fluff with a fork.

2. Put all the ingredients for the dressing into each jar, then whisk until combined.

3. Add your chosen protein option and carb option to the jar, then add the cucumber, red onion, tomatoes and lettuce. Now all you need to do is tip the jar upside down onto your plate! If the dressing gets stuck at the bottom of the jar, swirl a little water around the bottom of the jar to loosen it, then pour over the salad.

4. Store the jars in the fridge for up to 4 days.

Protein
17.5g

Serves: **4**   Prep time: **5 mins**   Cook time: **10 mins**
Cals: **491**   Carbs: **61.8g**   Protein: **17.5g**   Fat: **18.3g**

9 780241 693605

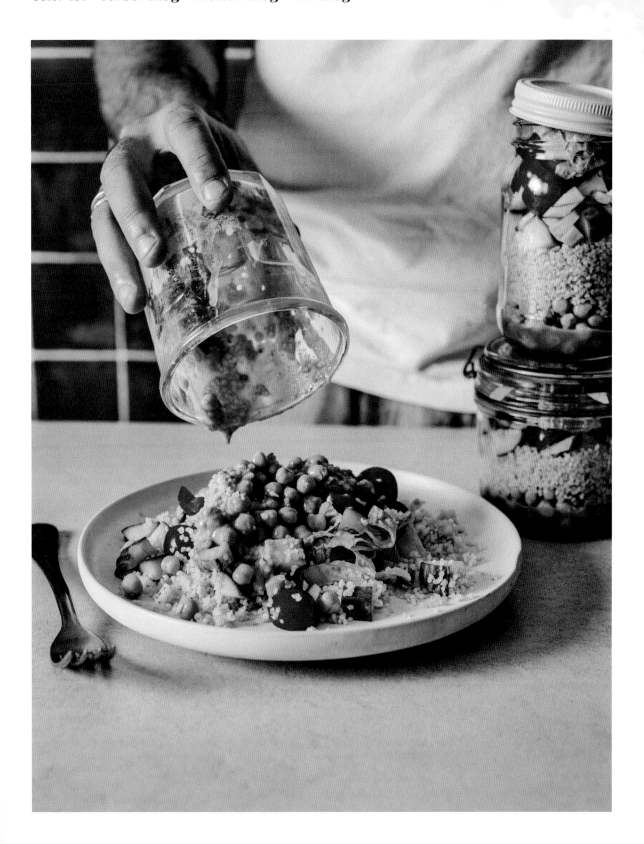

Avotuna Toasted Sandwiches

This is my version of Joe & the Juice's viral Tunacado sandwich. Pesto, sriracha mayonnaise, avocado, tomatoes and a delicious tuna mayo filling are all packed between two slices of toasted sourdough – there's a lot going on in this sandwich, but it's fresh, seriously tasty and perfect for lunchtime.

8 thin slices of sourdough bread
3 tbsp reduced-fat pesto
2 tbsp sriracha mayonnaise
1 large avocado, sliced
2 tomatoes, sliced

For the tuna filling

3 x 145g tins of tuna in spring
  water, drained
2 tbsp light mayonnaise
1 red onion, finely chopped
a bunch of fresh parsley,
  finely chopped
2–3 tbsp pickled jalapeños,
  finely chopped
2 tbsp jalapeño brine
juice of 1 lemon
salt and freshly ground
  black pepper

1. Mix together all the ingredients for the tuna filling in a large bowl.

2. Toast the bread, then spread half the slices with the pesto and drizzle with the sriracha mayonnaise. Add the tuna filling, then the avocado and tomato slices and close the sandwiches.

3. These will keep in the fridge for up to 4 days. Store in air tight containers, or wrap in tin foil or cling film and store in the fridge for up to 4 days.

Protein
27.3g

SANDWICHES & SALADS

Serves: **4**   Prep time: **5 mins**
Cals: **446**   Carbs: **52g**   Protein: **27.3g**   Fat: **14.7g**

9 780241 693612

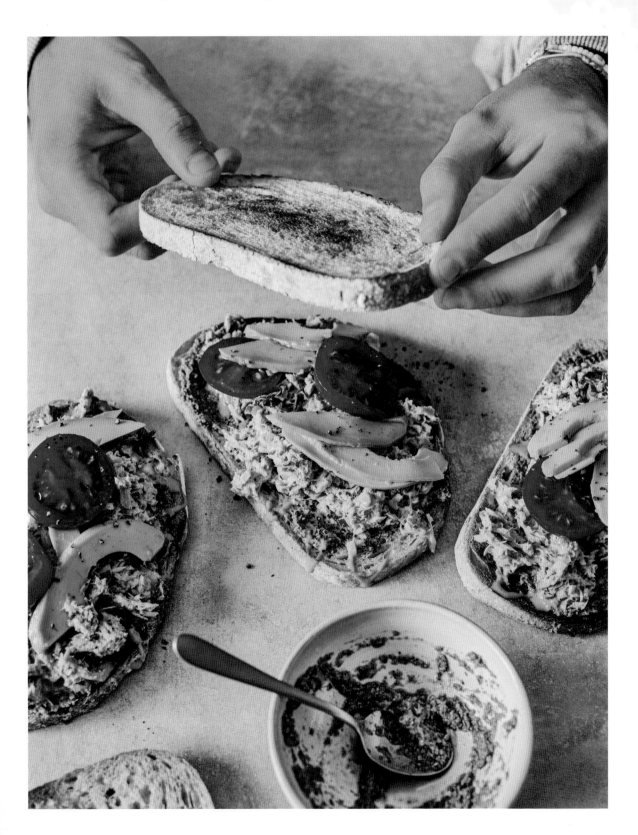

Serves: **4**   Prep time: **10 mins**   Cook time: **20 mins**
Cals: **447**   Carbs: **43.2g**   Protein: **30.6g**   Fat: **15.8g**

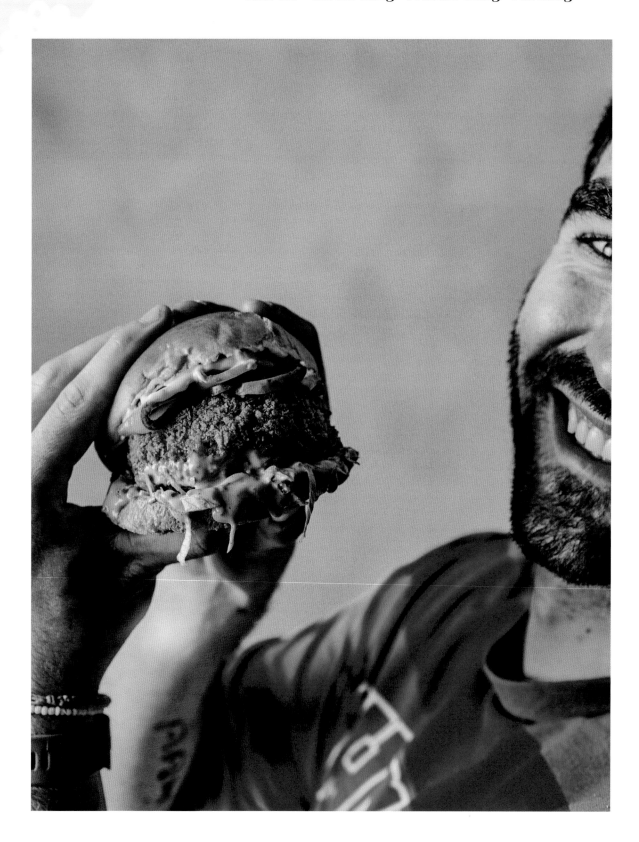

Crispy Chicken Sandwiches
WITH CHIPOTLE MAYO

These crispy chicken patties are spicy, but not too spicy. They're packed between toasted brioche buns with a chipotle mayo, lettuce and gherkins for maximum crunch. Using chicken mince for this recipe allows you to pack loads of seasoning into the patties, meaning you get bags of flavour with each bite. Coating chicken in cornflakes and baking is one of my favourite and most-used healthy cooking techniques because the chicken gets super crispy without the need for deep-frying.

For the patties

500g minced chicken
1 tsp onion granules
1 tsp garlic granules
1 tsp smoked paprika
1 tsp cayenne pepper
½ tsp salt
freshly ground black pepper

For the crispy coating

75g cornflakes
1 tsp smoked paprika
1 tsp cayenne pepper
½ tsp salt
2 egg whites
1 tbsp hot sauce
low-calorie cooking spray

To serve

6 tbsp light mayonnaise
1 tsp chipotle paste
4 brioche buns
iceberg lettuce, thinly sliced
2–3 sliced gherkins (optional)

1. Preheat the oven to 190°C (170°C fan/375°F/Gas 5).

2. Combine all the ingredients for the patties in a bowl and mix well to combine.

3. Put the cornflakes, smoked paprika, cayenne pepper and salt into a food processor and blend to a fine crumb, then pour onto a large plate.

4. Whisk together the egg whites and hot sauce in a bowl.

5. With wet hands, form the chicken mixture into four equal-sized patties. Dip the patties in the egg white mixture and then in the cornflake crumb, making sure they are coated all over. Spray with low-calorie cooking spray, then transfer to a baking sheet and bake in the oven for 15–20 minutes. Alternatively, cook in an air fryer at 200°C for 12–15 minutes.

6. Meanwhile, mix together half the mayonnaise with the chipotle paste in a small bowl.

7. Slice and toast the brioche buns and spread the bottom buns with the chipotle mayonnaise. Spread the top buns with the remaining mayonnaise. Top the bottom buns with the chicken patties, lettuce and gherkins, if using, then close to make burgers. Store in air tight containers, or wrap in tin foil or cling film and store in the fridge for up to 4 days.

Protein
30.6g

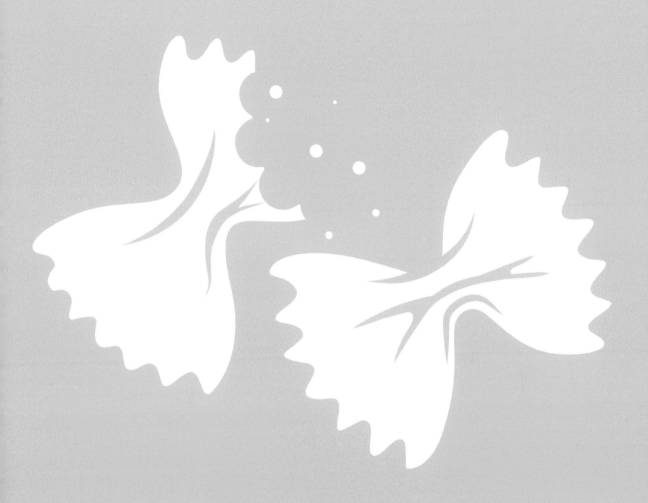

Perfect
Pastas

Baked Cajun Feta Orzo

This is a fuss-free, light, healthy and high-protein dish. All you need to do is chuck everything into a baking dish and bake it. The feta melts and combines with the sweet, jammy cherry tomatoes to create the perfect tangy and creamy sauce. Then all you have to do is shred the chicken breasts and throw in the orzo, and you have yourself the perfect meal prep. It's also great as it is delicious served both hot or cold.

3 small chicken breasts (400g)
150g block of full-fat feta cheese
½ tablespoon extra virgin olive oil
1 tablespoon Cajun seasoning
100g cherry tomatoes
300g orzo
a handful of spinach, roughly
  chopped
a handful of fresh basil,
  roughly chopped
salt and freshly ground
  black pepper

1. Preheat the oven to 180°C (160°C fan/350°F/Gas 4).

2. Put the whole chicken breasts and block of feta into a large baking dish, then drizzle with the oil. Sprinkle over the Cajun seasoning and rub into the chicken, then add the cherry tomatoes and bake in the oven for 20 minutes.

3. When there's 10 minutes of cooking time left, bring a large saucepan of salted water to the boil and cook the orzo until al dente. Drain, then rinse under cold water immediately.

4. Remove the baking dish from the oven and mash the baked feta and cherry tomatoes using a wooden spoon or fork. Shred the chicken breasts using two forks. Add the cooked orzo along with the spinach and basil, then mix until well combined. Season to taste before transferring to airtight containers. Store in the fridge for up to 4 days.

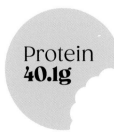

Protein
40.1g

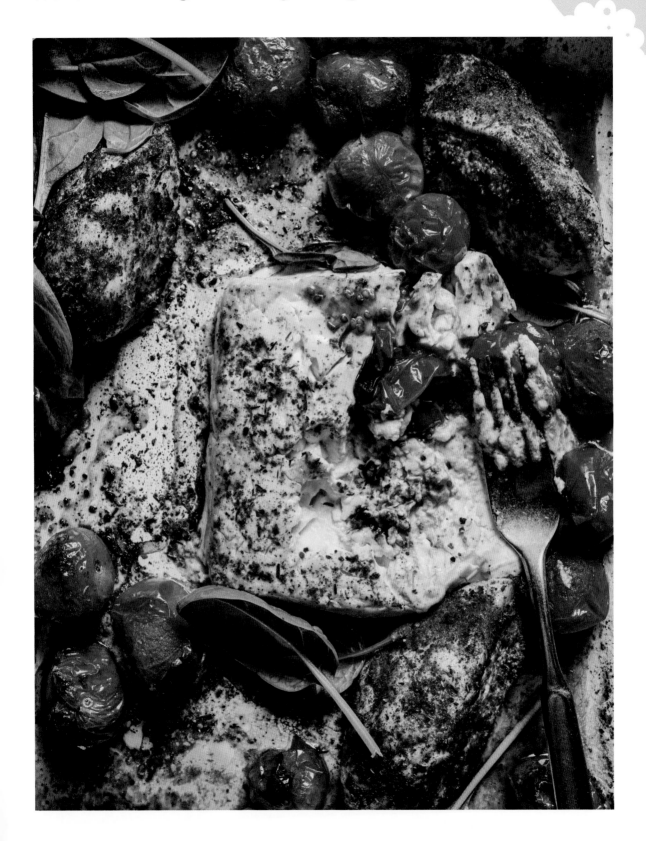

Serves: **4**   Prep time: **10 mins**   Cook time: **15 mins**
Cals: **440**   Carbs: **50.3g**   Protein: **31.6g**   Fat: **12.2g**

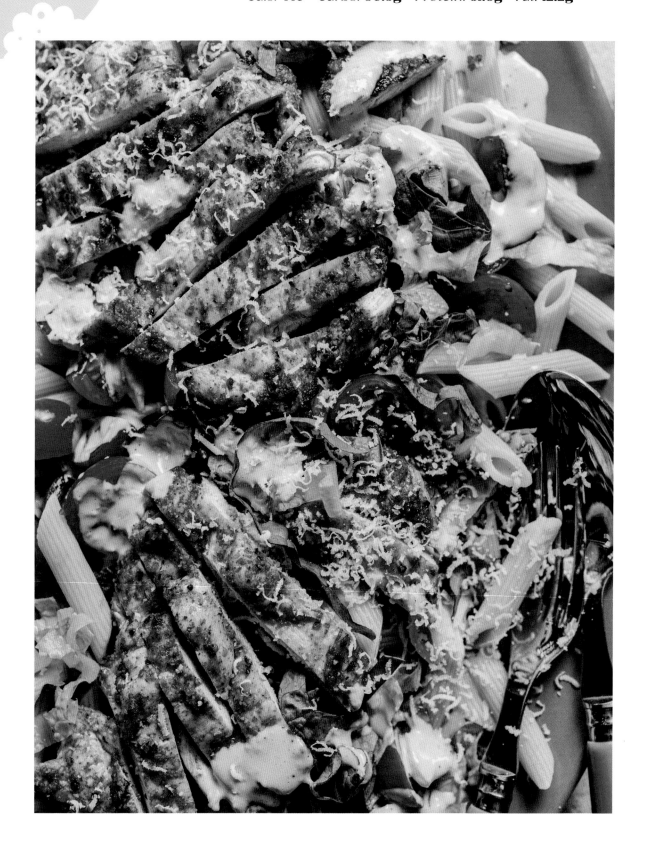

Chicken Caesar Pasta Salad

Calling all Caesar salad lovers! This recipe is a quick and easy Caesar pasta salad, using my delectable lighter Caesar dressing. It's served with spicy fried chicken breasts for a big hit of protein. This is the perfect meal prep for a hot summer's day.

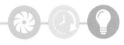

2 chicken breasts (400g)
1 tsp smoked paprika
1 tsp garlic granules
1 tsp onion granules
½ tsp dried oregano
½ tsp salt
½ tbsp extra virgin olive oil
250g penne, or similar pasta
200g cherry tomatoes
1 romaine lettuce, finely chopped

For the Caesar dressing

6 tbsp light mayonnaise
1 tsp anchovy paste
1 tsp Dijon mustard
1 clove of garlic, peeled and finely grated to make a paste
juice of 1 lemon
1 tsp Worcestershire sauce
1 tsp red wine vinegar
30g Parmesan, grated
freshly ground black pepper

1. Lay the chicken breasts flat on a board and butterfly them by slicing each one down the side to create four thinner breasts.

2. Coat the chicken breasts in the smoked paprika, garlic granules, onion granules, oregano, salt and extra virgin olive oil and cook in an air fryer at 190°C for 12–15 minutes. Alternatively, heat some oil in a non-stick frying pan and cook the chicken breasts for 5-10 minutes on each side, until cooked through.

3. Meanwhile, bring a large saucepan of water to the boil and cook the penne until dente, then drain and rinse under cold water.

4. Mix together the Caesar dressing ingredients in a bowl.

5. Slice the chicken, then transfer to a large bowl and add the pasta, tomatoes, lettuce and Caesar dressing. Mix until well combined.

6. Transfer to airtight containers and store in the fridge for up to 4 days.

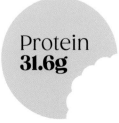

Protein
31.6g

Chicken Pesto Pasta Lunch Pots

I like a pasta pot for lunch, but the supermarket options are often underwhelming. These homemade pesto pasta pots solve that problem, and what makes them even better is that they're designed to be enjoyed cold! I've used shop-bought pesto and roasted chicken just to keep things as simple and quick as possible, but feel free to use homemade pesto or any leftover roast chicken you might have lying about in the fridge.

300g conchiglie, or similar pasta
150g pesto
75g fat-free Greek yoghurt
juice of ½ lemon
a handful of fresh basil, chopped
100g cherry tomatoes, halved
2 roasted red peppers (from a jar), chopped
20g pine nuts
20g Parmesan, shaved
30g rocket
300g roasted chicken breast, torn into fine pieces
salt

1. Bring a large saucepan of salted water to the boil and cook the conchiglie until al dente, then drain and rinse under cold water.

2. In a large bowl, whisk together the pesto, yoghurt and lemon juice, then add the pasta, basil, cherry tomatoes, roasted red peppers, pine nuts, Parmesan shavings and rocket. Finally, stir in the chicken.

3. Transfer to airtight containers and store in the fridge for up to 4 days.

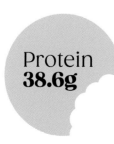

Protein
38.6g

Serves: **4**   Prep time: **5 mins**   Cook time: **10 mins**
Cals: **593**   Carbs: **59.7g**   Protein: **38.6g**   Fat: **21.4g**

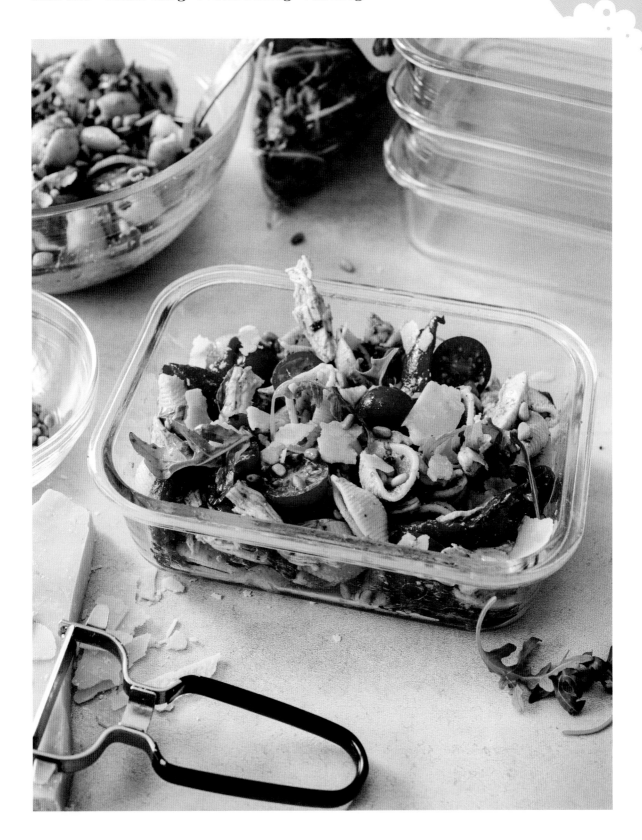

Cajun Chilli Prawn Linguine

This is a light and speedy recipe. Fiery king prawns are seasoned with Cajun spices and lime juice and served on a bed of linguine that has been tossed in a creamy, tomato and chilli sauce. Make this to please your family and friends at dinner or for an awesome make-ahead lunch for yourself.

1 tbsp extra virgin olive oil
3 cloves of garlic, peeled and
    finely chopped
2 small shallots, peeled and
    finely chopped
1 x 400g tin of chopped tomatoes
1 tbsp chilli purée
2 tbsp tomato purée
1 tsp smoked paprika
350g linguine
100ml single cream
75g Tenderstem broccoli, chopped
fresh basil, chopped
salt and freshly ground
    black pepper
20g Parmesan, grated, to serve

For the prawns

300g raw, peeled king prawns
½ tbsp Cajun seasoning
½ tbsp chilli purée
juice of 1 lime
1 red chilli, deseeded and finely
    chopped

1. First, marinate the prawns. Put the prawns into a bowl and toss with the Cajun seasoning, chilli purée, lime juice and chilli.

2. Heat the oil in a large non-stick saucepan over a high heat and cook the prawns for 5 minutes until pink, then remove from the pan and set aside.

3. Reduce the heat to medium-low and fry the garlic and shallots for 5 minutes until soft, then add the chopped tomatoes, chilli purée, tomato purée, smoked paprika and some salt and pepper. Stir well, then simmer for 10 minutes until thickened. For an extra smooth sauce, mash the tomatoes with a potato masher.

4. Meanwhile, bring a large saucepan of salted water to the boil and cook the linguine until al dente.

5. Add the single cream to the sauce along with the broccoli and a ladle of pasta water, then bring back to a low simmer and cook for 4–5 minutes until the broccoli is tender. Remove from the heat and add the pasta, basil and another ladle of pasta water. Toss to combine.

6. Transfer the linguine to airtight containers and top with the prawns and Parmesan. This will keep in the fridge for up to 4 days.

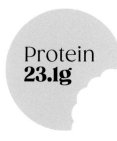

Protein
23.1g

Serves: **4**   Prep time: **5 mins**   Cook time: **25 mins**
Cals: **345**   Carbs: **36.8g**   Protein: **23.1g**   Fat: **11g**

87

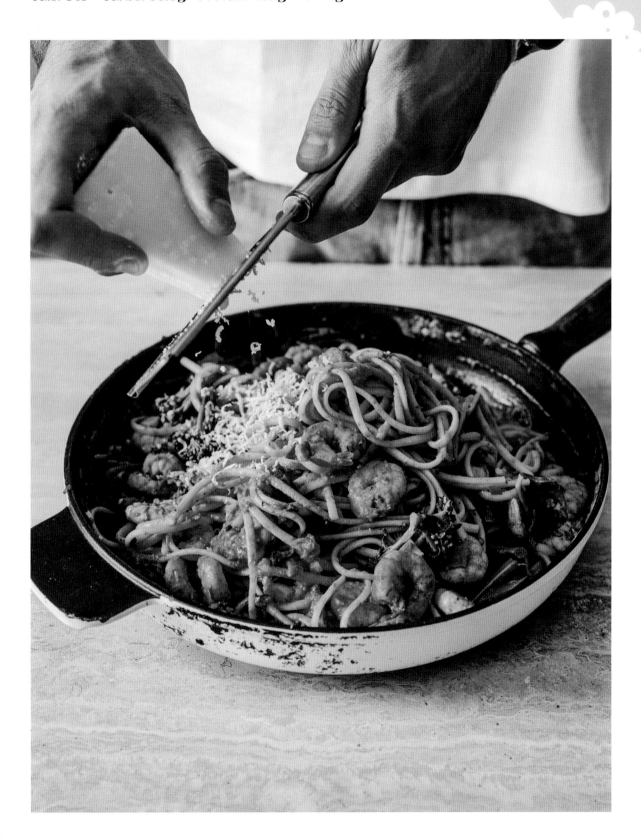

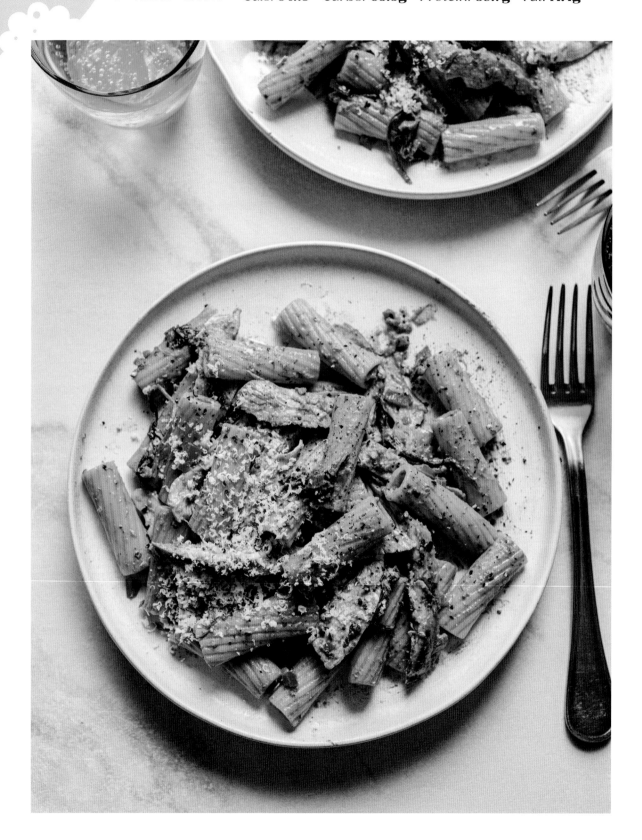

Creamy Peri-peri Rigatoni

Tasty and satisfying, yet so easy to make, this creamy and spicy pasta is an absolute winner. Best served hot.

2 chicken breasts (400g)
2 tbsp extra virgin olive oil
2 tbsp peri-peri seasoning
300g rigatoni
a splash of red wine vinegar (or any vinegar)
2 shallots, peeled and finely chopped
1 sweet Romano pepper, finely chopped
4 tbsp light cream cheese
3 tbsp tomato purée
1 tsp smoked paprika
1 tbsp dried oregano
a few handfuls of spinach
50ml single cream (optional)
30g Parmesan, grated, plus extra to serve

1. Place the chicken on a board, cover with cling film and use a rolling pin or mallet to flatten it to 2cm thick. Transfer to a bowl and coat with 1 tablespoon of the olive oil and 1 tablespoon of the peri-peri seasoning.

2. Bring a large saucepan of salted water to the boil and cook the rigatoni until al dente, then drain, reserving the pasta water in a jug or bowl.

3. Meanwhile, heat the remaining tablespoon of olive oil in a large, deep frying pan or saucepan over a medium heat, then add the chicken. Fry for 4–5 minutes on each side until slightly charred and cooked through, then remove from the pan.

4. Deglaze the pan with the red wine vinegar, then add the shallots and Romano pepper. Fry for 5 minutes over a low-medium heat, stirring occasionally, before adding the cream cheese, tomato purée, the remaining tablespoon of peri-peri seasoning, smoked paprika, oregano and a large ladle of pasta water, creating a creamy sauce. Stir in the spinach, single cream, if using, and cooked rigatoni. Once the spinach has wilted, remove the pan from the heat. Add the Parmesan and more pasta water if needed.

5. Thinly slice the chicken breasts, then transfer the pasta and chicken to airtight containers and finish with a little more grated Parmesan. This will keep for up to 4 days.

Protein
39.7g

9 780241 693681

Serves: **4**   Prep time: **10 mins**   Cook time: **25 mins**
Cals: **583**   Carbs: **76.5g**   Protein: **43.6g**   Fat: **11.2g**

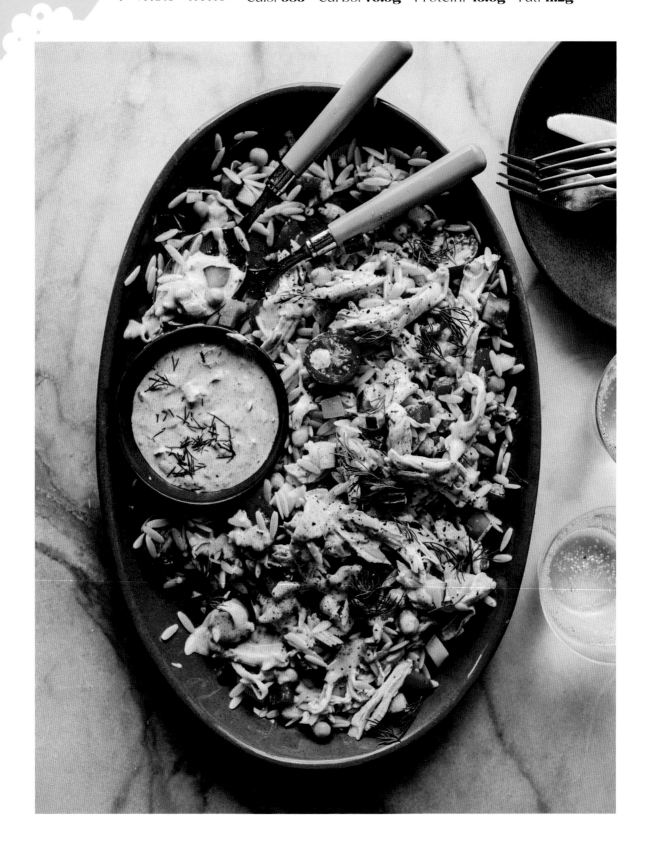

Creamy Garlic Chicken & Orzo Pasta Salad

This is one of the creamiest, most indulgent salads you'll have ever made. It's packed with protein and perfect for easy meal prep. It's something to look forward to for lunch or even a light summer dinner.

2 chicken breasts (400g)
½ tbsp extra virgin olive oil
2 cloves of garlic, peeled
   and crushed
1 tbsp dried oregano
350g orzo
2 peppers (any colour), finely
   chopped
½ red onion, finely chopped
½ small cucumber, deseeded and
   finely chopped
125g cherry tomatoes, halved
120g drained and rinsed chickpeas
salt and freshly ground
   black pepper

For the creamy dressing

150g fat-free natural yoghurt
2 tbsp light mayonnaise
1 tsp Dijon mustard
1 tsp garlic granules
1 tsp smoked paprika
1 tbsp extra virgin olive oil
juice of 1 lemon
a small handful of fresh dill,
   roughly chopped
half a bunch of fresh parsley,
   roughly chopped

1. Preheat the oven to 190°C (170°C fan/375°F/Gas 5).

2. Put the chicken breasts into a baking dish with the olive oil, garlic, oregano and some salt and pepper. Stir to coat, then bake in the oven for 20–25 minutes. Alternatively, cook in an air fryer at 200°C for 15–20 minutes.

3. Meanwhile, bring a large saucepan of salted water to the boil and cook the orzo until al dente, then drain and rinse under cold water.

4. Combine all the creamy dressing ingredients in a bowl and mix well.

5. Once cooked, cut or shred the chicken into small pieces, then transfer to a large bowl with the pasta, remaining ingredients and the dressing. Toss well to combine.

6. Transfer to airtight containers and store in the fridge for 3–4 days.

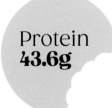

Protein
43.6g

Cajun Garlic Parmesan Alfredo

This is one of the most popular recipes on the website and across our social media channels. It's a lighter, high-protein twist on a classic Alfredo. The double cream-based sauce is swapped out for one made with semi-skimmed milk and light cream cheese, and the addition of Cajun spices creates a delicious garlicky, herby and cheesy pasta sauce that takes this dish to the next level. You won't believe how well it works until you try it for yourself.

4 small chicken breasts
(450–500g)
1 tbsp extra virgin olive oil
2 tbsp Cajun seasoning, or more
to taste
20g unsalted butter
1 onion, chopped
3 cloves of garlic, peeled and
finely chopped
300ml semi-skimmed milk
3 tbsp light cream cheese
200ml hot chicken stock
300g linguine, or similar pasta
75g Parmesan, grated
1 tsp dried parsley
freshly ground black pepper
fresh parsley, chopped, to garnish

1. Preheat the oven to 190°C (170°C fan/375°F/Gas 5).

2. Put the chicken breasts into a large baking dish with the oil and 1 tablespoon of the Cajun seasoning. Stir to coat, then bake in the oven for 25 minutes. Alternatively, cook in an air fryer at 200°C for 15–20 minutes.

3. Meanwhile, heat the butter in a large saucepan over a medium heat and fry the onion for 5 minutes until softened, then add the garlic and fry for a further 2 minutes.

4. In a bowl or jug, whisk together the milk and cream cheese, then add to the pan along with the chicken stock. Simmer aggressively for 15 minutes, stirring regularly, until reduced by half. If the milk starts to bubble over, reduce the heat so that it doesn't catch on the bottom.

5. Bring a large saucepan of salted water to the boil and cook the linguine until very al dente (around 8 minutes), then drain, reserving the pasta water. Rinse the pasta under cold water until completely cooled, then fill the pan with cold water and place the pasta back in the saucepan.

6. Once the sauce has reduced and is a nice, thick, creamy consistency, stir in the remaining Cajun seasoning and remove from the heat. Add the Parmesan, dried parsley and plenty of black pepper, then stir to combine.

7. Transfer a small amount of the sauce to sauce pots for pouring over, then drain the pasta and add it to the pan along with a ladle of the pasta water. Toss to combine over a medium heat, adding more pasta water if needed.

8. Divide the pasta into airtight containers. Slice the chicken and add to the pasta, then garnish with fresh parsley. This will keep in the fridge for up to 4 days.

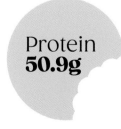

Protein
50.9g

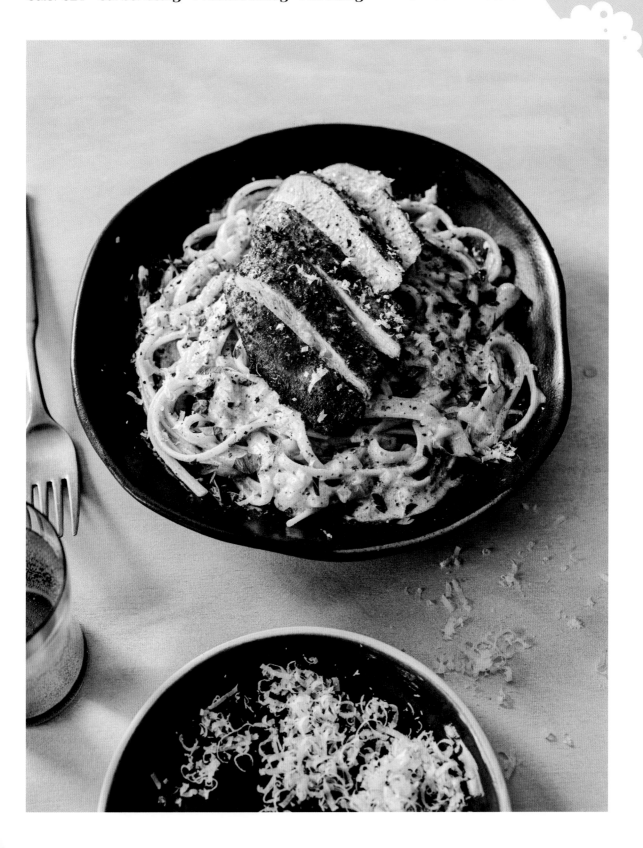

9 780241 693704

Serves: **4**   Prep time: **5 mins**   Cook time: **25 mins**

Cals: **685**   Carbs: **59.4g**   Protein: **38.2g**   Fat: **31.9g**

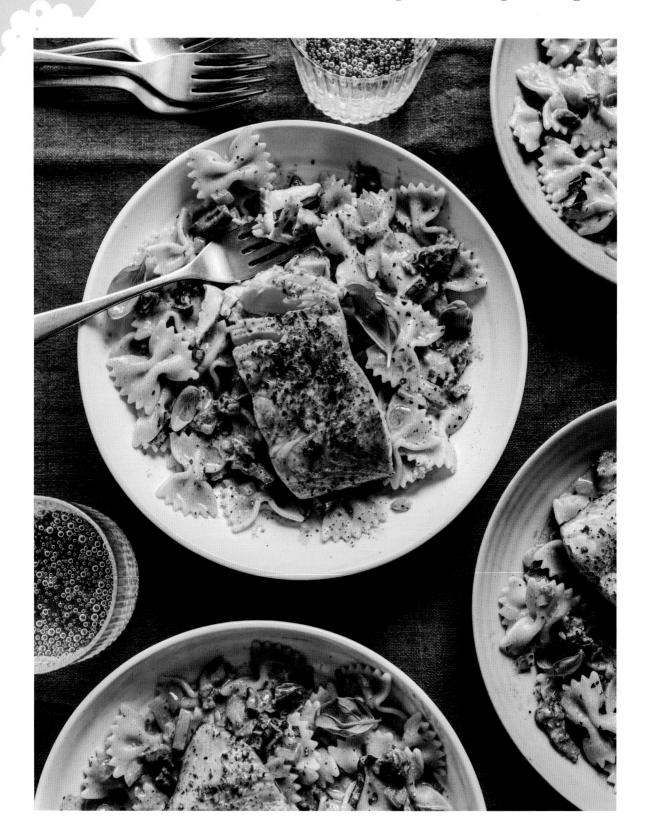

Creamy Sun-dried Tomato & Salmon Pasta

Salmon fillets pan-fried in sun-dried tomato oil, with sautéed onion and garlic serving as the base to a creamy but light pasta sauce with hints of smoked paprika and fresh basil. I love this recipe and it's so easy to knock up and be ready in 30 minutes. It's designed as a banging meal prep, but would also work perfectly to serve to family or friends as an impressive weeknight dinner.

1 tbsp sun-dried tomato oil (from the jar)
4 x 110g salmon fillets
½ tsp chilli flakes, plus a pinch for each salmon fillet
½ tbsp dried oregano, plus extra for the salmon
1 onion, finely chopped
3 cloves of garlic, peeled and crushed
300g farfalle
100g sun-dried tomatoes, drained and chopped
250ml vegetable stock
75ml single cream
½ tsp smoked paprika
a small bunch of fresh basil, leaves picked
20g Parmesan, grated, plus extra to serve
salt and freshly ground black pepper

1. Heat the sun-dried tomato oil in a large, non-stick frying pan over a medium heat, then season the salmon fillets with a little salt, pepper, chilli flakes and oregano and place skin side down in the pan. Cook for 3–4 minutes on each side until the skin is crispy and the salmon is cooked through, making sure the skin doesn't catch and stick to pan. Remove from the pan and set aside.

2. Put the onion and garlic into the pan and fry over a low heat for 5 minutes, stirring regularly.

3. Meanwhile, bring a large saucepan of salted water to the boil and cook the pasta until al dente, then drain, reserving a ladle of the pasta water.

4. Add the sun-dried tomatoes and vegetable stock to the onions and bring to a low simmer, then stir in the smoked paprika, oregano and chilli flakes and cook for 5–10 minutes until thickened.

5. Stir in the cream and basil, then remove from the heat and stir in the Parmesan. Once combined, add the pasta and a ladle of pasta water and toss until you have a glossy sauce.

6. If eating straight away, place the salmon on top of the pasta and cover with a lid to allow the salmon to reheat for 2–4 minutes.

7. Otherwise, transfer the pasta to airtight containers and place the salmon fillets on top. This will keep in the fridge for up to 4 days.

Protein
38.2g

Air Fryer Lasagne

One day I had the crazy idea to try to make lasagne in an air fryer, and it came out perfect!
This recipe makes four perfectly sized portions and bakes in a fraction of the time it takes to bake
a lasagne in the oven. It still hits the spot just like a traditional lasagne, with a rich beef ragu
layered between pasta sheets with a white sauce, all topped with gooey melted cheese.
On top of all that, it's only 430 calories per portion!

500g lean minced beef (5% fat)
2 cloves of garlic, peeled and
   finely chopped
1 onion, peeled and finely chopped
1 stick of celery, chopped
400g passata
1 tbsp red wine vinegar
1 tsp dried oregano
a handful of fresh basil, chopped
8–10 lasagne sheets
300g white sauce (homemade or
   shop-bought; I used Heinz)
50g reduced fat mozzarella
   cheese, greated
15g Parmesan, grated
low-calorie cooking spray
salt and freshly ground
   black pepper

For the white sauce:

50g butter
50g plain flour
600ml whole milk
50g Cheddar cheese
salt and black pepper, to season

1. Heat a few sprays of low-calorie cooking spray in a large, non-stick saucepan over a medium heat and cook the beef for 3–4 minutes until browned all over, then add the garlic, onion and celery and cook for 4 minutes.

2. Add the passata, red wine vinegar, oregano and basil and simmer for 10 minutes.

3. Line an air fryer basket with baking paper and add a layer of the beef sauce, then add a layer of lasagne sheets, then a layer of white sauce. Repeat until everything is used up, reserving some white sauce for the top. Finish with the mozzarella and Parmesan.

4. If you'd like to make your own white sauce, melt the butter in a saucepan. Then add the plain flour and stir continuously until it turns into a roux - a paste. Add the milk to the roux, stirring continuously again until you have a creamy sauce. Finally add the seasoning and Cheddar Cheese and stir.

5. Cook in the air fryer at 170°C for 15 minutes and check with a knife to see if tender. If you notice that the top layer is getting too crisp, cover with foil and continue cooking. Leave the lasagne to rest for 10 minutes before slicing into four slices.

6. Transfer to airtight containers and store in the fridge for up to 4 days.

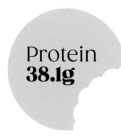

Protein
38.1g

Serves: **4**   Prep time: **5 mins**   Cook time: **35 mins**
Cals: **430**   Carbs: **44.3g**   Protein: **38.1g**   Fat: **10.8g**

97

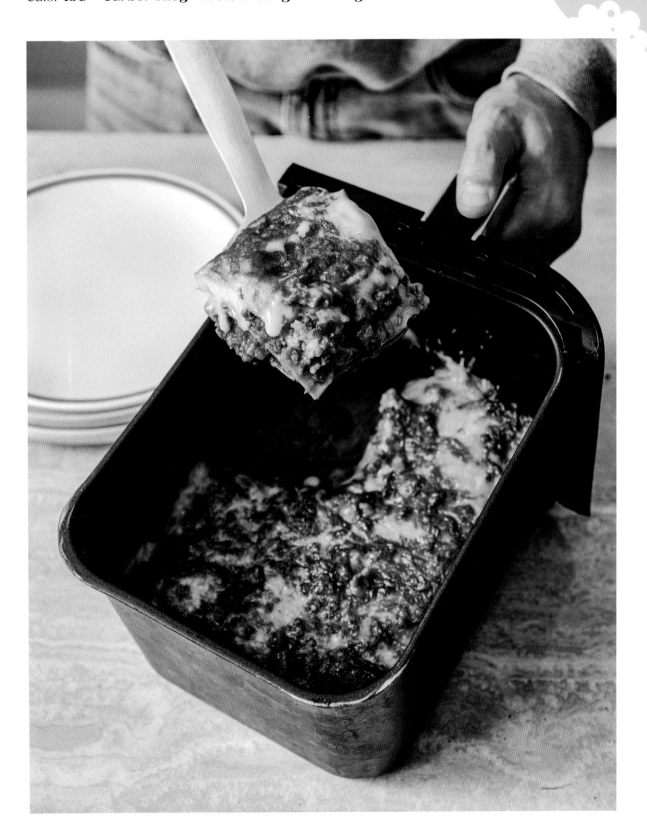

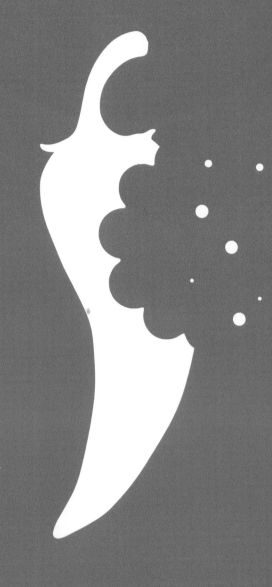

Noodles
& Rice

Serves: **4**   Prep time: **5 mins**   Cook time: **25 mins**

With chicken: Cals: **563**   Carbs: **89.2g**   Protein: **39.1g**   Fat: **5.3g**

With king prawns: Cals: **511**   Carbs: **89.2g**   Protein: **27.5g**   Fat: **4.7g**

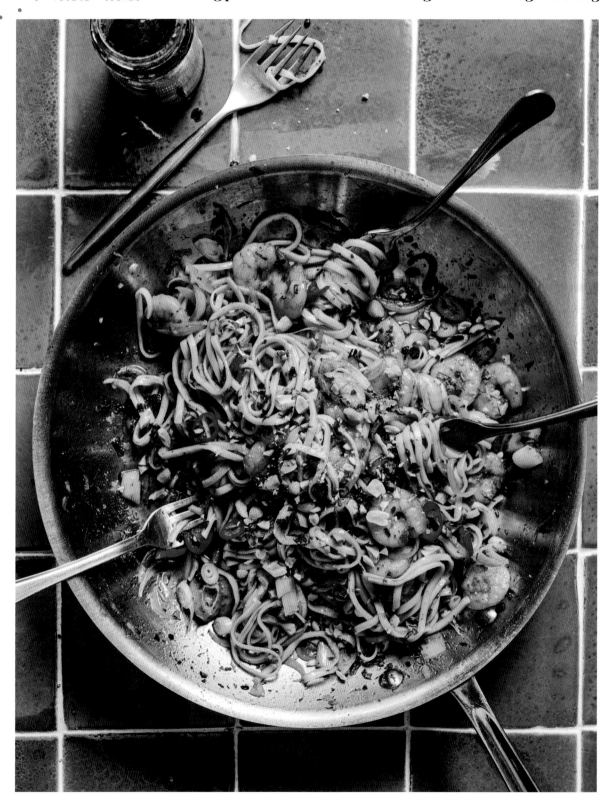

Chilli Oil Noodles
WITH GARLIC CHICKEN OR PRAWN BITES

Spicy chilli oil noodles with tender, garlicky chicken or prawns make a banging meal prep recipe that takes only 15 minutes to cook. This version has been adapted from a popular recipe on the website – all you need to do is season and fry the chicken, sauté the aromatics, mix the sauce and then chuck it all together. It couldn't be simpler. Best served hot.

400g dried udon noodles
2 small onions, thinly sliced
2 cloves of garlic, peeled
  and grated
10g fresh ginger, peeled
  and grated
4–5 spring onions, finely chopped
1–2 red chillies, deseeded and
  thinly sliced
3 tbsp light soy sauce
2 tbsp runny honey
1½ tbsp crispy chilli oil

For the chicken or prawn bites
450g chicken breast, diced, or
  350g raw, peeled king prawns
½ tbsp garlic granules
½ tbsp onion granules
½ tbsp smoked paprika
½ tbsp groundnut oil

To serve
1 red chilli, deseeded and finely
  chopped
1 spring onion, finely chopped
fresh coriander, chopped
a handful of whole blanched
  peanuts, finely chopped

1. In a bowl, mix together the chicken or prawns, garlic granules, onion granules and smoked paprika.

2. Bring a large saucepan of water to the boil and add the noodles. Cook according to the packet instructions, then drain and add to a large bowl of cold water to stop the cooking process. Set aside in the water while you cook everything else.

3. Heat the oil in a large, non-stick frying pan over a medium heat and add the chicken or prawns. For chicken, cook for 5 –10 minutes until charred on the outside and cooked through, then remove from pan and set aside. For prawns, cook for 3–4 minutes until pink, then remove from the pan and set aside.

4. Reduce the heat and add the onion to the pan. Cook for 3-4 minutes until soft, then add the garlic, ginger, spring onions and chilli and cook for 2 minutes, stirring regularly.

5. Add the cooked noodles and chicken or prawns to the pan along with the soy sauce, honey and crispy chilli oil, then toss to combine.

6. Transfer to airtight containers and garnish with the chilli, spring onion, coriander and peanuts. Store in the fridge for up to 3 days.

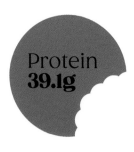

Protein
39.1g

Aromatic Chilli Beef Noodles

I came up with this recipe because I wanted to see if I could adapt the classic takeaway crispy chilli beef into a fuss-free meal prep option. I've fried the beef in aromatics, Chinese five spice, soy sauce and honey to achieve that distinctive flavour and then coupled it up with a simple noodle stir-fry. The result is a sumptuous bowl of noodles that is high in protein and perfect for your packed lunch. Best served hot.

For the noodles

200g dried egg noodles
½ tbsp groundnut oil
2 shallots, peeled and finely chopped
1 red pepper, roughly chopped
3–4 spring onions, roughly chopped
100g Tenderstem broccoli, roughly chopped
a handful of kale, roughly chopped
1 tbsp light soy sauce
1 tbsp dark soy sauce
2 tbsp mirin
½ tbsp sesame oil
2 tbsp ketjap manis (sweet soy sauce)
1 tbsp sriracha
a few leaves of pak choi, thinly sliced lengthways

For the beef

½ tbsp groundnut oil
3 cloves of garlic, peeled and finely chopped
20g fresh ginger, peeled and finely chopped
1 tsp chilli flakes
400g lean minced beef (5% fat)
1 tsp onion granules
2 tsp Chinese five spice
1 tbsp dark soy sauce
1 tbsp runny honey

To serve

sesame seeds
fresh coriander, chopped

1. Bring a large saucepan of water to the boil and cook the noodles according to the packet instructions, then drain and rinse under cold water.

2. Meanwhile, make the beef. Heat the oil in a large, non-stick frying pan or wok over a low heat and add the garlic, ginger and chilli flakes. Fry for 2–3 minutes until fragrant, then add the beef and cook for 5 minutes, breaking it up with a wooden spoon or spatula, until browned. Add the onion granules, Chinese five spice, soy sauce and honey, then cook for a further 3–4 minutes. Once the beef has soaked up the soy sauce and honey, remove from the pan and set aside.

3. Next, make the noodles. Wipe out the pan with kitchen paper, then heat the oil over a low-medium heat and stir-fry the shallots and pepper for 2 minutes. Add the spring onions, broccoli and kale and fry for a further 2 minutes, then add the noodles, light soy sauce, dark soy sauce, mirin, sesame oil, ketjap manis, sriracha, pak choi and half the chilli beef. Toss well until combined.

4. Transfer the noodles to airtight containers and top with the remaining aromatic beef, then sprinkle with the sesame seeds and coriander. This will keep in the fridge for up 4 days.

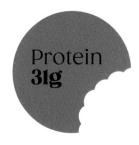

Protein
31g

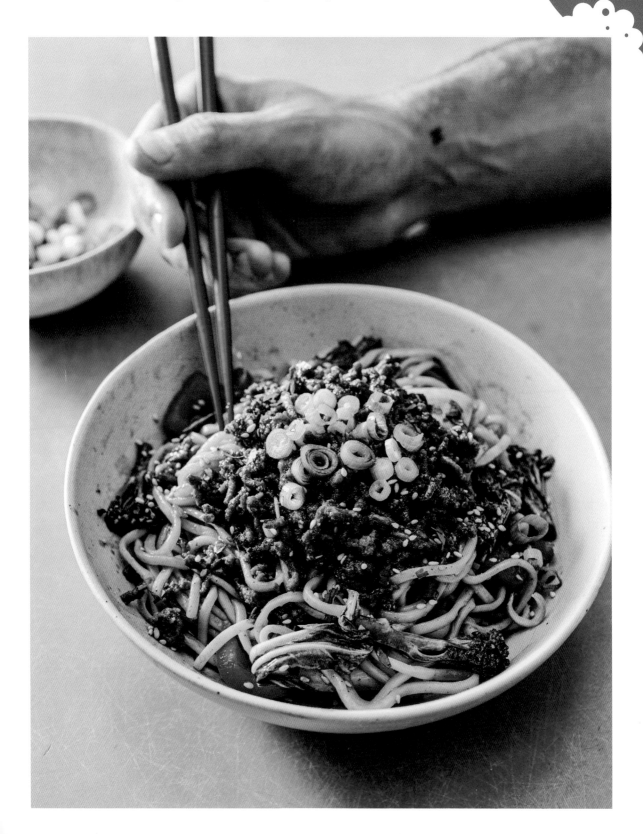

Creamy Peanut Noodles
WITH PRAWNS

This is one of the easiest and simplest recipes in the whole book, but the flavour in these creamy peanut noodles is unbelievable! All you need to do is cook the noodles and mix together that simple peanut sauce, then chuck it all together in a big bowl with the cooked prawns. Simple, healthy, high in protein and delicious. It can also be served hot or cold.

200g dried egg noodles
100g mangetout
300g cooked, peeled prawns
3–4 spring onions, thinly sliced
lime wedges, to serve

For the peanut sauce

2 tbsp dark soy sauce
2 tbsp rice wine vinegar
1–2 tbsp sriracha, depending on
  spice preference
1 tbsp sesame oil
6 tbsp crunchy peanut butter
2 tbsp runny honey
3 cloves of garlic, peeled and
  finely grated
4cm piece of fresh ginger, peeled
  and finely grated
1 large red chilli, deseeded and
  finely chopped

1. Bring a large saucepan of water to the boil and cook the noodles according to the packet instructions, then drain, reserving some of the cooking water.

2. Steam the mangetout in a steamer for 2–3 minutes until cooked but still crunchy.

3. In a large bowl, mix together the peanut sauce ingredients with 4 tablespoons of the reserved noodle water.

4. Add the noodles to the peanut sauce along with the prawns, mangetout and spring onions, then toss to combine.

5. Transfer to airtight containers and add the lime wedges, then store in the fridge for 3–4 days.

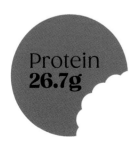

Protein
26.7g

Serves: **4**   Prep time: **5 mins**   Cook time: **10 mins**

Cals: **437**   Carbs: **49.9g**   Protein: **26.7g**   Fat: **14g**

9 780241 693742

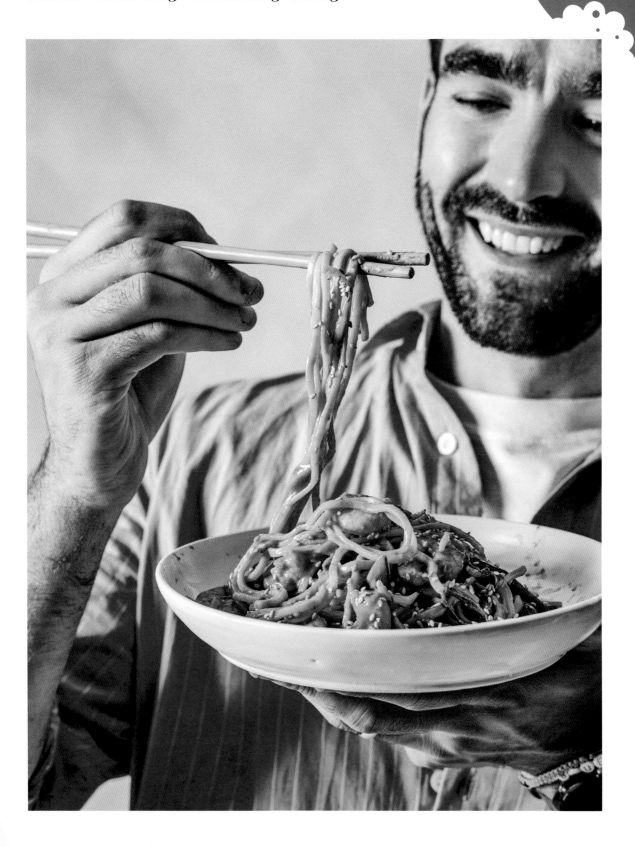

9 780241 693759

Serves: **4**   Prep time: **5 mins**   Cook time: **15 mins**
Cals: **477**   Carbs: **47.7g**   Protein: **45.1g**   Fat: **11.6g**

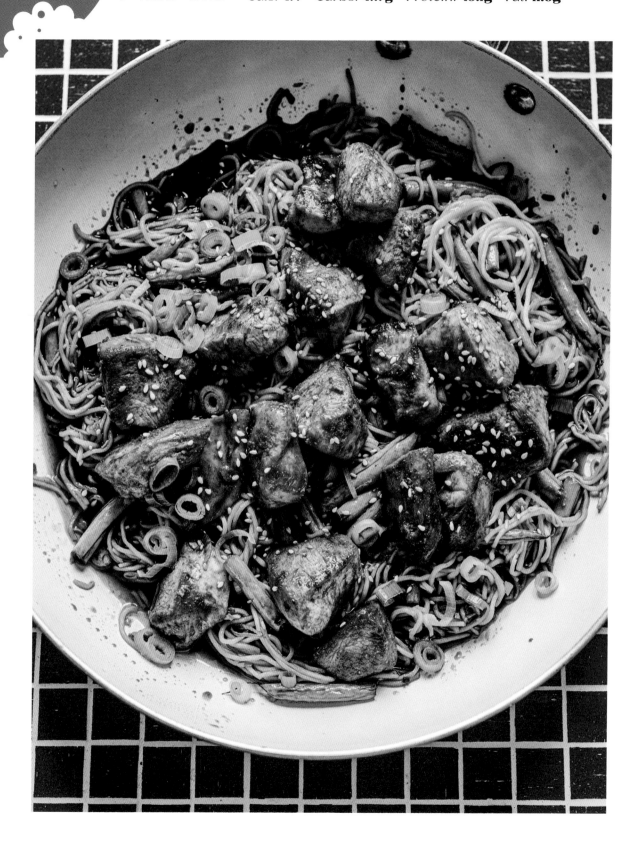

Spicy honey-garlic Chicken Noodles

Yes, there is a lot of garlic in this recipe … It may be best to pack this meal on days when you don't have back-to-back meetings! Either way, it's a delicious, easy and high-protein noodle dish that will keep you fuelled throughout the day. When you combine the noodles with the sauce, be careful not to keep the pan on the heat for too long so that it doesn't become stodgy.

600g chicken breast, diced
200g dried fine egg noodles
1 tbsp groundnut oil
5 cloves of garlic, peeled and finely chopped
4 spring onions, separated into white and green parts, then finely chopped
100g green beans, thinly sliced lengthways
low-calorie cooking spray
sesame seeds, to garnish

For the marinade

1 tbsp groundnut oil
1 tbsp dark soy sauce
2 cloves of garlic, peeled and finely chopped
1½ tsp smoked paprika
½ tsp cayenne pepper
salt and freshly ground black pepper

For the sauce

2 tbsp light soy sauce
2 tbsp dark soy sauce
1 tbsp rice wine vinegar
3 tbsp runny honey
1–2 tbsp sriracha

1. In a bowl, whisk together all the ingredients for the marinade. Add the chicken and stir to coat.

2. In a separate bowl, whisk together the sauce ingredients.

3. Bring a large saucepan of water to the boil and cook the noodles according to the packet instructions, then drain.

4. Meanwhile, heat a few sprays of low-calorie cooking spray in a large non-stick frying pan and fry the chicken for 5–7 minutes until cooked through and slightly charred, then remove from the pan.

5. Heat the oil in the pan, then reduce the heat to low and add the garlic and the white parts of the spring onions. Fry for 2 minutes, then add the green beans. Fry for a further 2 minutes, then add the sauce along with the noodles. Toss to combine until the noodles are coated. There should be enough oil to stop the noodles sticking, but if they do seem sticky, then add a splash of groundnut or sesame oil before boxing up.

6. Transfer the noodles to airtight containers and top with the chicken. Garnish with the green parts of the spring onions and the sesame seeds. This will keep in the fridge for 3–4 days.

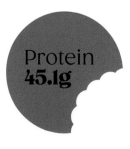

Protein
45.1g

Serves: **4**   Prep time: **5 mins**   Cook time: **20 mins**
Cals: **626**   Carbs: **79.9g**   Protein: **53.9g**   Fat: **9.5g**

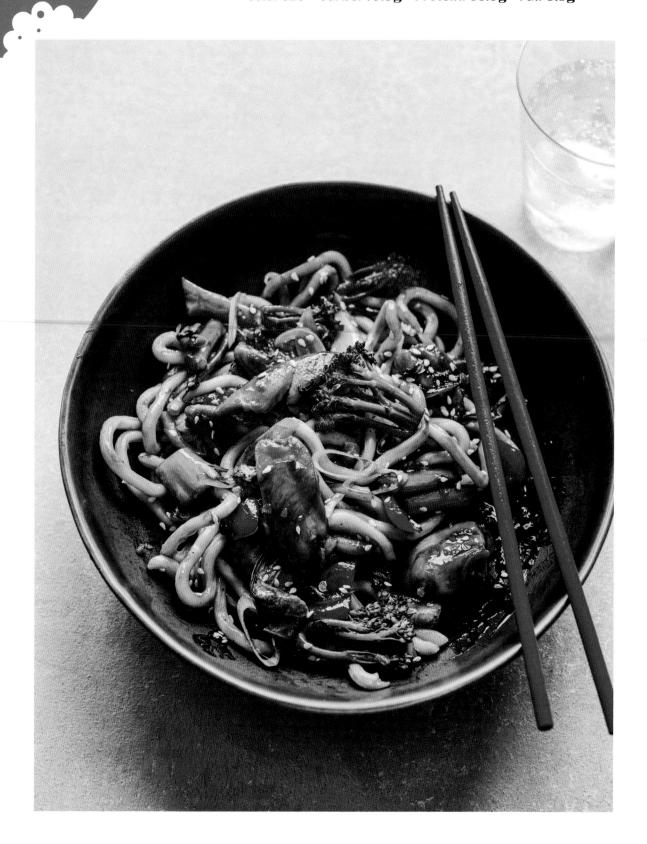

Teriyaki Noodles

These teriyaki noodles are a healthy, high-protein and delicious meal prep option that are ready in just 20 minutes. Staying on track with your diet doesn't need to be difficult or boring, and I've added the option of king prawns for a slightly lower calorie option, too. Reserve some of that delicious teriyaki sauce to drizzle over the noodles just before eating. Best served hot.

500g boneless, skinless chicken thighs, thickly sliced, or 300g raw, peeled king prawns
½ tbsp groundnut oil
1 onion, thinly sliced
1 red pepper, roughly chopped
100g Tenderstem broccoli, roughly chopped
600g straight-to-wok udon noodles
4 spring onions, roughly chopped
1 pak choi, thinly sliced
salt and freshly ground black pepper
sesame seeds, to garnish

For the sauce
80ml dark soy sauce
80ml mirin
3 tbsp runny honey
1 tsp groundnut oil
2 cloves of garlic, peeled and finely chopped
4cm piece of fresh ginger, peeled and finely chopped
1 tbsp cornflour, mixed into a slurry with 2 tbsp water

1. First, make the sauce. In a bowl, whisk together the dark soy sauce, mirin and honey. Heat the oil in a frying pan over a low heat, then add the garlic and ginger. Fry for 2–3 minutes until softened, stirring regularly, then add the soy sauce mixture. Bring to a gentle simmer, then cook for 2 minutes. Add the cornflour slurry, stir well and allow the sauce to come back to a simmer. Once the sauce starts bubbling and thickens, remove from the heat and add half of the sauce to sauce pots, reserving the rest to add to the noodles later.

2. Season the chicken or prawns all over with salt and pepper. Heat the oil in a non-stick frying pan over a medium heat and fry the chicken for 5–10 minutes until cooked through, then remove from pan. If using prawns, cook for 3–4 minutes until pink, then remove from the pan.

3. Add the onion, red pepper and broccoli to the pan and stir-fry for 3 minutes until charred but still crunchy.

4. Add the chicken or prawns back to the pan along with the noodles, spring onions, pak choi and remaining teriyaki sauce. Toss to combine, then transfer to airtight containers and sprinkle with the sesame seeds. This will keep in the fridge for up to 4 days.

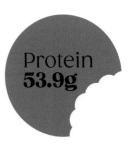

Protein
53.9g

Crispy Chilli Beef Noodle Salad

This is a 'healthier than takeaway' fakeaway that I have adapted into a noodle salad to work as a meal prep option. I've made it as low-calorie as possible without losing the crispiness and intense flavour that we all love crispy chilli beef for. The noodle salad is light and crunchy and thrown together in a matter of minutes.

2 egg whites
1 tbsp soy sauce
1 tsp Chinese five spice
400g lean beef strips
100g cornflour
1 tbsp groundnut oil
200g dried egg noodles
½ tbsp sesame oil
juice of 1 lime
1 tbsp sriracha
1 red pepper, thinly sliced
1 carrot, thinly sliced
a handful of radishes, chopped
4 spring onions, thinly sliced on
 the diagonal
2 red chillies, sliced, to garnish
sesame seeds, to garnish

For the chilli sauce

1 tbsp soy sauce
4 tbsp reduced-sugar sweet
 chilli sauce
2 tbsp ketchup
3 tbsp runny honey
1 tbsp tomato purée
4 tbsp rice wine vinegar
1 clove of garlic, peeled and
 finely grated
1 thumb-sized piece of fresh
 ginger, finely grated

1. Mix together all the ingredients for the chilli sauce in a bowl, then set aside.

2. Whisk the egg whites, soy sauce and Chinese five spice in a large bowl, then add the beef strips, and massage the marinade into the beef.

3. Put the cornflour into a large Tupperware box, then add the beef, seal the box and shake vigorously until the beef strips are coated in cornflour.

4. Transfer the beef to an air fryer basket and toss with the groundnut oil, then cook at 200°C for 10 minutes until crispy. Alternatively, heat the oil in a non-stick frying pan and fry the beef until crispy.

5. Bring a large saucepan of water to the boil and add the noodles, then turn off heat and leave the noodles to soak for 5–6 minutes. Drain and rinse under cold water, then transfer to a large bowl and toss with the sesame oil. Add half the chilli sauce, the lime juice, sriracha, red pepper, carrot, radishes, spring onions (reserving some for garnishing) and toss to combine.

6. Combine the crispy beef and remaining chilli sauce in a large saucepan and cook over a medium heat, tossing together, for 2-4 minutes, until the sauce thickens and coats the beef.

7. Divide the noodle salad among airtight containers and top with the crispy chilli beef, then garnish with the reserved spring onions, the red chilli and sesame seeds.

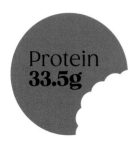

Protein
33.5g

Serves: **4**   Prep time: **4 mins**   Cook time: **15 mins**
Cals: **549**   Carbs: **79.5g**   Protein: **33.5g**   Fat: **11.4g**

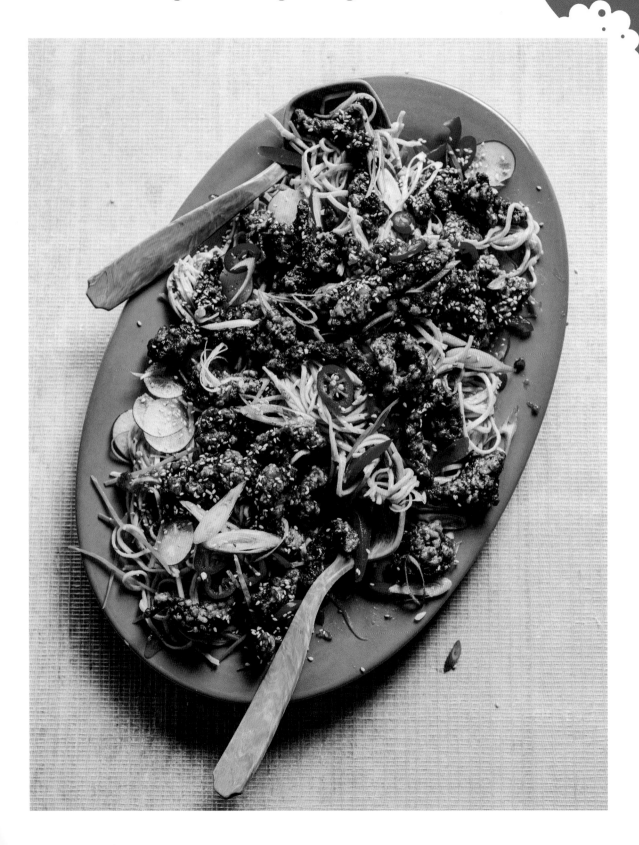

Serves: **4**   Prep time: **5 mins**   Cook time: **12 mins**
With chicken: Cals: **430**   Carbs: **45.5g**   Protein: **30.5g**   Fat: **13.7g**
With tofu: Cals: **432**   Carbs: **47.3g**   Protein: **24.4g**   Fat: **15.7g**

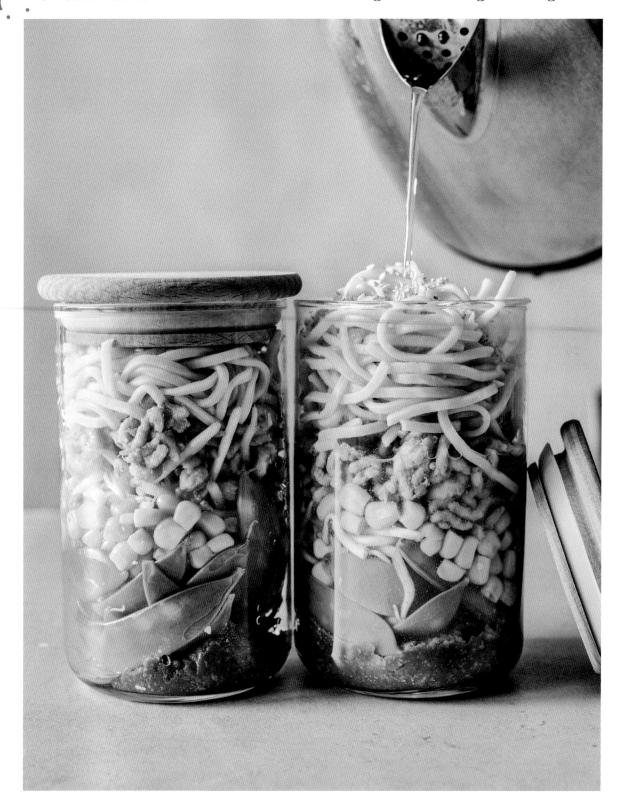

Miso Ramen Noodle Jar

These noodle jars are one of those meal-prep hacks that will bring a smile to your face. Simply pack your chicken or tofu into jars along with miso paste, noodles and vegetables and store in the fridge. Then, all you need to do is add boiling water, give it a stir and tip it all out into a bowl. There's not many things more satisfying than serving yourself a perfect bowl of mouth-watering ramen in minutes. Best served hot.

200g dried egg noodles

1 tbsp sesame oil

400g minced chicken or 1 x 450g
  block of firm tofu, crumbled

2 cloves of garlic, peeled
  and crushed

15g fresh ginger, grated

1 tbsp soy sauce

2 tbsp red miso paste

100g mangetout

150g sweetcorn kernels

200g bean sprouts

20g sesame seeds

2 spring onions, thinly sliced

2 hard-boiled eggs (optional)

chilli oil (optional)

salt and freshly ground
  black pepper

1. Bring a large saucepan of water to the boil and cook the noodles for 3 minutes, then drain and rinse under cold water.

2. Heat the sesame oil in a non-stick frying pan over a medium heat, then add the chicken or tofu, garlic, ginger and salt and pepper and cook for 5 minutes, breaking up the chicken with a spoon, until browned. Add the soy sauce and cook for 3 minutes until it has been absorbed.

3. Divide the red miso paste among four jars, then add the mangetout, sweetcorn, bean sprouts, meat or tofu, noodles and sesame seeds. Put the spring onions, boiled eggs and chilli oil, if using, into separate containers. Seal the jars and store in the fridge for up to 4 days.

4. Before eating, allow the jar to come to room temperature for 10 minutes before adding boiling water and stirring well. Pour the contents of the jar into a bowl and garnish with the spring onions, eggs and chilli oil.

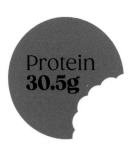

Protein
30.5g

Satay Chicken Rice Box

This satay sauce is just impossible not to love! It's rich and creamy and the red Thai curry paste really helps to take the flavours to a different level. Pack it into sauce pots and drizzle it over the juicy marinated chicken skewers, brown rice and crunchy vegetables when serving. Best served hot.

For the satay sauce

100g crunchy peanut butter
2 tbsp red Thai curry paste
200ml reduced-fat coconut milk
1 tbsp dark soy sauce
1 tbsp rice wine vinegar
½ tbsp runny honey
a handful of fresh coriander,
    finely chopped

For the chicken skewers

500g chicken breast, diced
1 tbsp red Thai curry paste
1 tbsp curry powder
juice of ½ lime
low-calorie cooking spray,
    for frying

To serve

300g brown rice
½ red cabbage, thinly sliced
1 small cucumber, sliced diagonally
4 lime wedges
15g blanched peanuts, chopped

1. Bring a large saucepan of water to the boil and cook the rice according to the packet instructions, then drain.

2. Meanwhile, make the satay sauce base. Mix together the peanut butter, curry paste, half the coconut milk, the soy sauce and rice wine vinegar in a medium bowl.

3. In a separate bowl, combine all the ingredients for the chicken skewers and add half the satay sauce base. Stir well until the chicken is coated. Thread the chicken pieces onto eight skewers, then spray all over with low-calorie cooking spray. Cook in an air fryer at 200°C for 12 minutes or pan-fry for 10 minutes until the chicken is cooked through.

4. Meanwhile, pour the remaining satay sauce base into a saucepan and add the remaining coconut milk, the honey and 150ml water. Stir to combine, then bring to a low simmer and cook until the sauce thickens. Stir in the coriander and transfer to sauce pots.

5. Transfer the rice and satay skewers to airtight containers, then add the red cabbage, cucumber and lime wedges. Garnish with the chopped peanuts. This will keep in the fridge for up to 4 days.

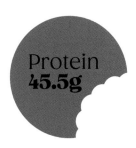

Protein
45.5g

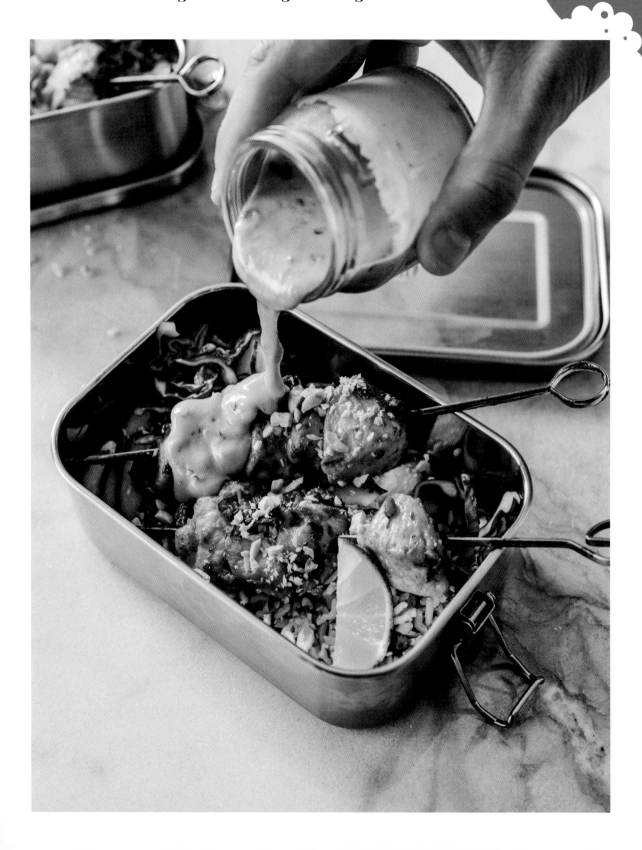

Bang Bang Salmon Rice Bowl

This homemade bang bang sauce is sweet, creamy and spicy. It can be used as a drizzle or dip in so many different recipes, but it's perfect with these amazing air-fried salmon bites. Best served hot.

4 x 120g salmon fillets, cut into
   large pieces
½ teaspoon sesame oil
1 tbsp BBQ seasoning
½ tbsp garlic granules

For the bang bang sauce
4 tbsp light mayonnaise
4 tbsp reduced-sugar sweet
   chilli sauce
1½ tbsp sriracha

To serve
240g sticky jasmine rice
150g edamame
2 carrots, julienned
100g radishes, thinly sliced
150g leafy green salad
sesame seeds

1. Preheat the oven to 200°C (180°C fan/400°F/Gas 6) and line a baking tray with baking paper.

2. Bring a large saucepan of water to the boil and cook the rice according to the packet instructions, then drain.

3. Meanwhile, put the salmon pieces into a bowl and toss with the sesame oil, BBQ seasoning and garlic granules. Transfer to the prepared baking tray and bake in the oven for 10 minutes. Alternatively, cook in a lined air fryer at 180°C for 8 minutes.

4. Whisk together the bang bang sauce ingredients with 2 tablespoons water and transfer to sauce pots.

5. Transfer the rice and salmon bites to airtight containers and add the edamame, carrots, radishes and salad. Garnish with sesame seeds. This will keep in the fridge for up to 4 days.

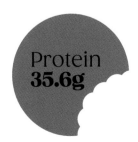

Protein
35.6g

Serves: **4**   Prep time: **5 mins**   Cook time: **15 mins**

Cals: **669**   Carbs: **63.8g**   Protein: **35.6g**   Fat: **31g**

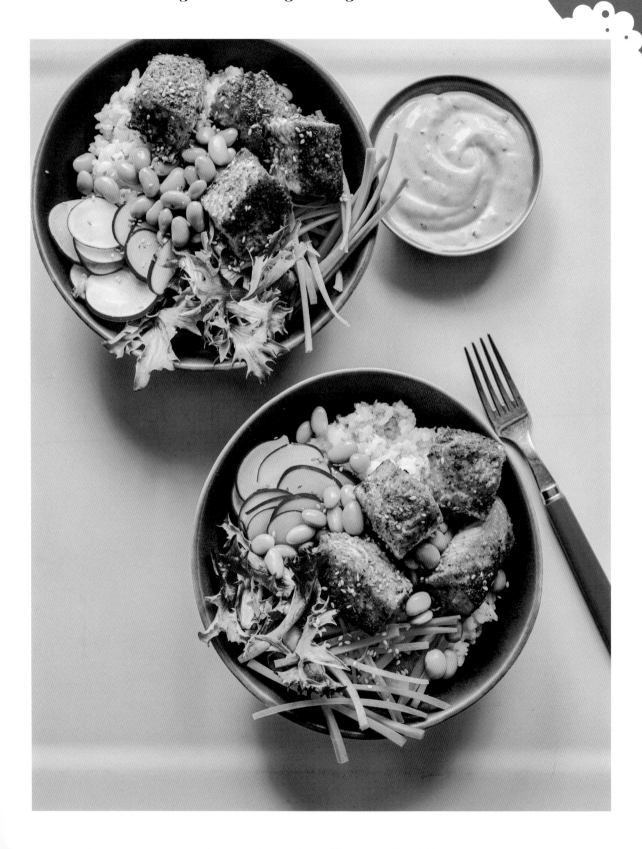

Serves: **4**   Prep time: **5 mins**   Cook time: **35 mins**

Cals: **605**   Carbs: **73.3g**   Protein: **37.7g**   Fat: **18.7g**

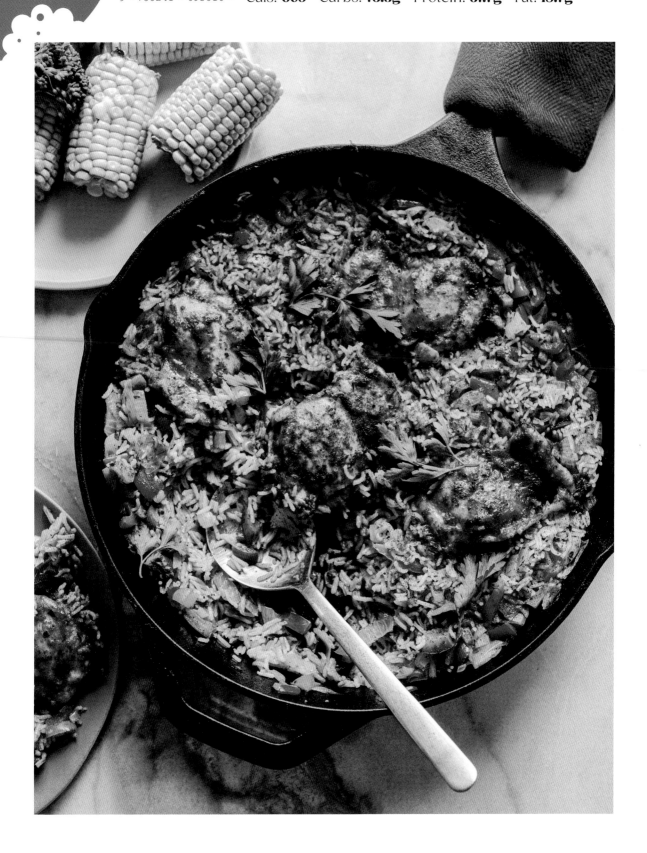

Peri-peri Rice Bake
WITH GRILLED CORN

Rice bakes are so easy but pack so much flavour. For this one, all you need to do is sear the chicken thighs, briefly cook the vegetables and then chuck in the rice. What you'll be left with is juicy peri-peri chicken, crunchy veg and flavourful rice that has soaked up all the lovely spices and seasoning. This recipe got over three million views on The Good Bite Instagram page and people loved it! I've adapted it slightly to make it more of a meal prep recipe by adding grilled corn and broccoli.

500g boneless, skinless chicken thighs
1 tbsp extra virgin olive oil
2 tbsp peri-peri spice rub or seasoning
1–2 tbsp peri-peri sauce
1 onion, finely chopped
2 peppers (any colour), finely chopped
250g basmati rice, rinsed
1 tsp smoked paprika
1 tbsp dried parsley
500ml hot chicken stock
4 corn on the cobs
1 tbsp reduced-fat butter spread
100g Tenderstem broccoli
fresh parsley, chopped, to serve

1. Preheat the oven to 180°C (160°C fan/350°F/Gas 4).

2. Put the chicken thighs, half the olive oil, 1 tablespoon of the peri-peri spice rub and 1 tablespoon of the peri-peri sauce into a large bowl and stir to coat.

3. Heat the remaining oil in a cast-iron frying pan or ovenproof casserole dish over a high heat and add the chicken thighs. Cook for 3–4 minutes on each side until cooked through. Brush the thighs with a little more peri-peri sauce, then remove from the pan and reduce the heat to low.

4. Add the onion and peppers to the pan and fry for 5 minutes until soft. Add the rice, the remaining tablespoon of peri-peri spice rub, the smoked paprika and dried parsley, then increase the heat to medium. Toast the rice with the seasonings for 1–2 minutes, stirring constantly, then add the hot chicken stock. Bring everything to a rapid simmer, stir well, then add the chicken thighs back into the pan on top of the rice. Cover the pan with a lid or tightly wrap in tin foil, then bake in the oven for 15–20 minutes. When cooked, the rice should be fluffy, with no excess liquid in the pan.

5. While the rice bake is baking, wrap the corn in cling film and microwave for 4 minutes on high. Unwrap and brush with the butter, then transfer to a frying pan or cast-iron griddle and cook over a high heat for 4–6 minutes until charred. Alternatively, cook in an air fryer at 200°C for 6–8 minutes, or wrap in tin foil and roast the corn in the oven for 35 minutes.

6. Steam the broccoli in a steamer for 3–4 minutes until cooked but still with a little bite.

7. Remove the rice from the oven and garnish with the parsley. Transfer to airtight containers along with the corn and broccoli. This will keep in the fridge for 3–4 days.

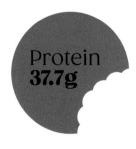

Protein
37.7g

Honey BBQ Beef Fried Rice

A simple fried rice recipe that packs in a tonne of flavour. The honey BBQ sauce gives this dish an Asian-American fusion feel and delivers a wonderfully sweet, tangy and smoky flavour profile. This is ready in 30 minutes and is best served hot.

400g lean minced beef (5% fat)
1 tsp garlic granules
1 tsp onion granules
½ tbsp BBQ seasoning
½ tbsp groundnut oil
1 onion, thinly sliced
1 green pepper, diced
150g mixed frozen vegetables
2 x 250g packets of basmati
   microwave rice
2 spring onions, thinly sliced
1 tbsp dark soy sauce
a squeeze of lime juice
1 tbsp sriracha (optional)
low-calorie cooking spray
salt and freshly ground
   black pepper

For the honey BBQ sauce
4 tbsp BBQ sauce
3 tbsp runny honey
1 tbsp soy sauce
2 tbsp rice wine vinegar
1 tbsp tomato purée

1. Mix together all the ingredients for the honey BBQ sauce in a bowl, then set aside.

2. Heat a few sprays of low-calorie cooking spray in a large, non-stick frying pan over a high heat and cook the beef for 5 minutes until browned all over. Add the garlic granules, onion granules and BBQ seasoning and some salt and pepper. Stir to combine, then reduce the heat to low and add half the honey BBQ sauce. Toss until the beef is coated with the sauce, then remove from the pan.

3. Heat the groundnut oil in the same pan and add the onion and pepper. Cook for 2–3 minutes until starting to soften, then add the mixed frozen vegetables, rice, spring onions (reserving some for garnishing) and soy sauce. Stir-fry for 3–4 minutes over a high heat, then add the remaining sauce (reserving 2 tablespoons to drizzle over when serving), half the beef, a squeeze of lime and the sriracha, if using. Stir-fry for 3–4 minutes, then remove from the heat.

4. Divide the rice among airtight containers and top with the reserved beef. Garnish with the reserved spring onions and sauce. Keep in the fridge for 3–4 days.

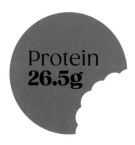

Protein
26.5g

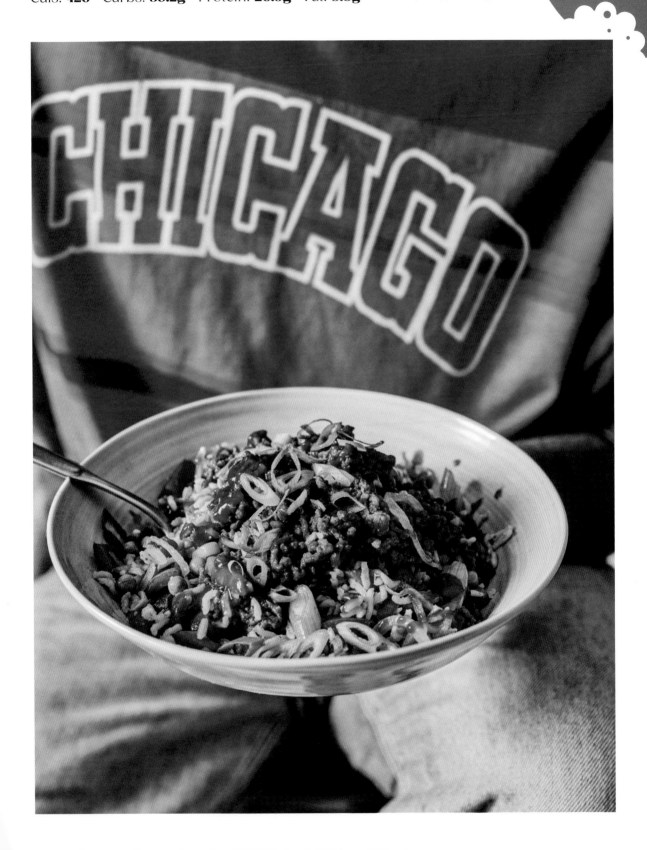

Aioli Chicken Rice Box

Juicy grilled chicken thighs, coupled up with a creamy, garlicky aioli, brown rice and pomegranate seeds, creating the perfect mouthful with every bite – meal prep doesn't get much better than this! When making the aioli for these rice boxes, I first infuse the lemon juice with the garlic to avoid that overpowering flavour that can come from raw garlic. Don't worry, it still has a great garlicky flavour, but if you do love that powerful garlic taste, just skip that step and add the garlic straight to the rest of the aioli ingredients. These were inspired by the popular high-street lunch chain, Leon.

300g brown rice
500g boneless, skinless
  chicken thighs
1½ tsp garlic granules
juice of 1 lemon
1 tbsp extra virgin olive oil
salt and freshly ground
  black pepper

For the aioli

5 cloves of garlic, peeled and
  grated into a paste
juice of ½ lemon
100g fat-free Greek yoghurt
60g light mayonnaise
a pinch of fine sea salt
a pinch of freshly ground
  black pepper
¼–½ tsp Dijon mustard

To serve

50g pomegranate seeds
sumac
lemon wedges

1. Bring a large saucepan of water to the boil and cook the rice according to the packet instructions, then drain and cover.

2. Meanwhile, make the aioli. Combine the garlic and lemon juice in a shallow bowl and leave to sit 10 minutes, allowing the lemon juice to soak up the flavour from the garlic. Place a fine sieve over a bowl, then pour the lemon juice and garlic into the sieve and press through using a rubber spatula or spoon, allowing the garlicky lemon juice to drip into the bowl. Add the remaining aioli ingredients with 50ml cold water and mix until combined, then transfer to sauce pots.

3. Put the chicken into a bowl and add the garlic granules, lemon juice and some salt and pepper. Heat the oil in a cast-iron griddle or frying pan over a medium heat and cook the chicken for 5 minutes on each side until cooked through and charred.

4. Transfer the rice and chicken to airtight containers, then garnish with the pomegranate seeds, sumac and lemon wedges. Store in the fridge for up to 4 days.

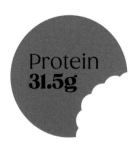

Protein
31.5g

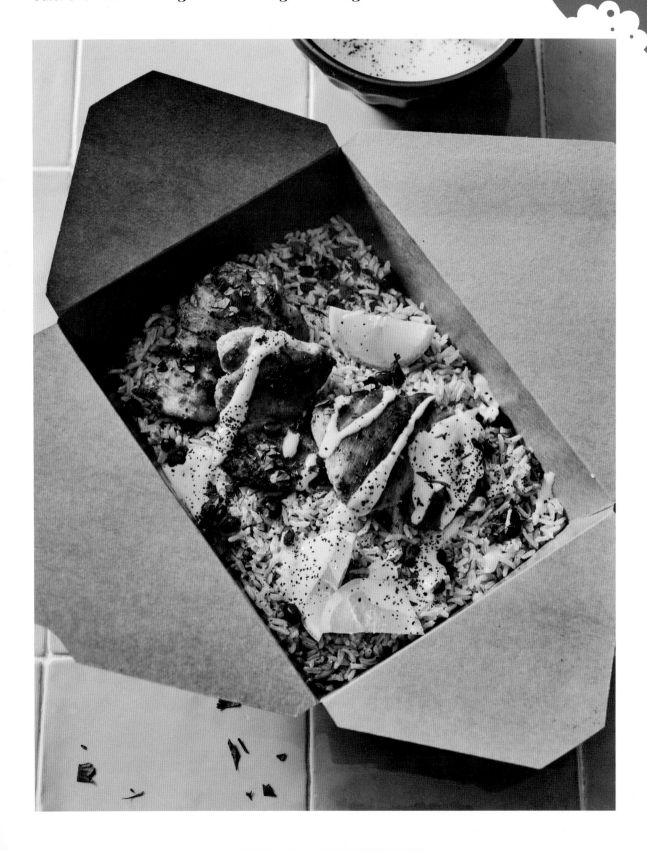

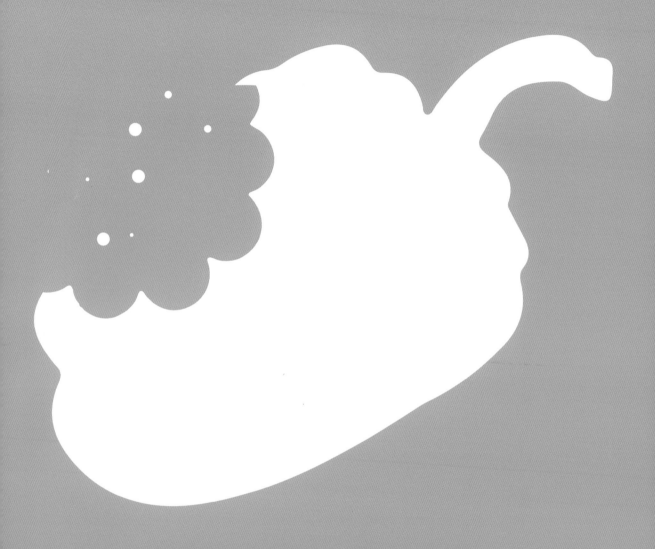

Weeknight Feasts

Prosciutto-stuffed Chicken Breasts
WITH CRISPY PESTO POTATOES

I love this recipe because of how easy and fuss-free it is to make. The chicken breast is stuffed with garlicky and herby cream cheese and wrapped in prosciutto to keep it juicy and full of flavour. The potatoes just need seasoning and baking or air frying until crispy, then toss them in pesto. Easy, light and healthy!

60g light cream cheese

3 cloves of garlic, peeled and crushed

2 tbsp finely chopped fresh parsley

4 small chicken breasts (125g each)

8 slices of prosciutto

freshly ground black pepper

rocket salad, to serve

For the crispy potatoes

3 x 400g tins of peeled new potatoes in water or 750g new potatoes, peeled and chopped

½ tbsp extra virgin olive oil

1 tsp smoked paprika

1 tsp dried parsley

1 tsp salt

50g pesto

1. Preheat the oven to 200°C (180°C fan/400°F/Gas 6).

2. First, make the potatoes. Drain and rinse the potatoes under cold water, then pat dry with kitchen paper before transferring to a large bowl.

3. Coat in the olive oil, smoked paprika, dried parsley and salt, then transfer to a baking tray and bake in the oven for 35–40 minutes until crispy. Alternatively, cook in an air fryer at 200°C for 25 minutes. Once baked, transfer back to the bowl and toss with the pesto. Next, make the chicken.

4. Mix together the cream cheese, garlic and parsley in a bowl and season with pepper.

5. Slice the chicken breasts horizontally and stuff with the garlic and herb cream cheese, then wrap two slices of prosciutto around each chicken breast.

6. Place on a baking tray and bake in the oven for 20–25 minutes. Alternatively, cook in an air fryer at 200°C for 15 minutes.

7. Transfer to airtight containers and serve with the rocket salad. This will keep in the fridge for up to 4 days.

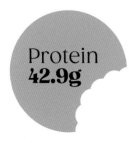

Protein
42.9g

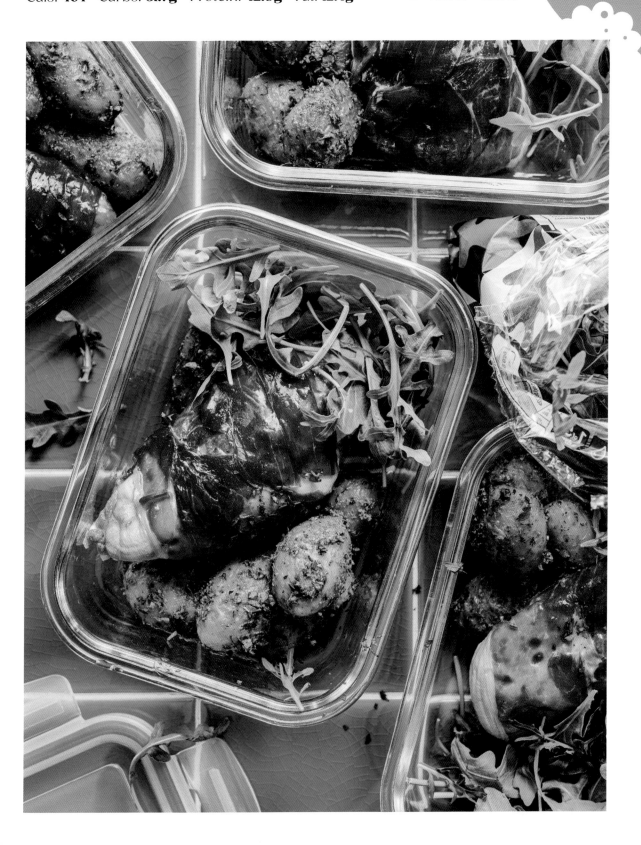

Serves: **4**   Prep time: **10 mins**   Cook time: **30 mins**
Cals: **532**   Carbs: **55.3g**   Protein: **43.2g**   Fat: **15.2g**

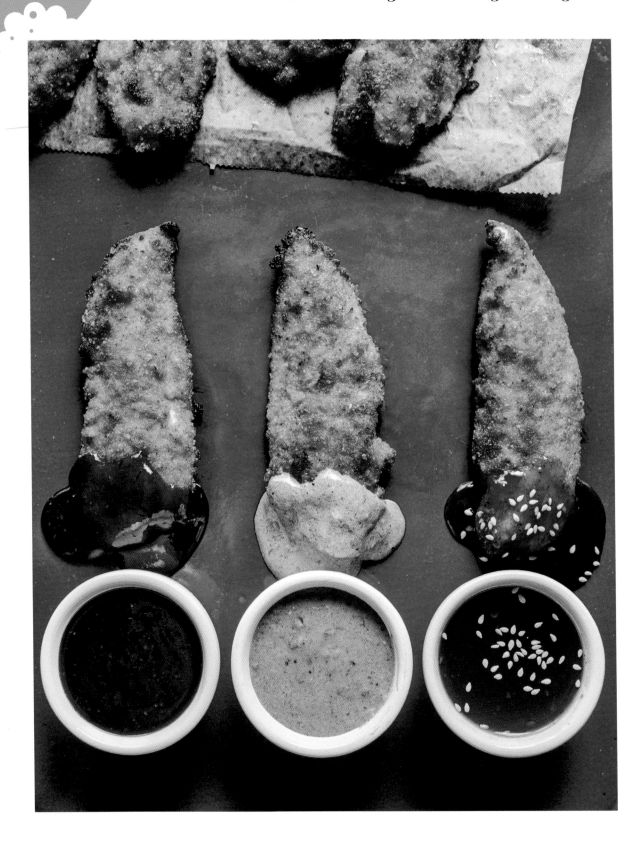

Chicken Tenders
THREE WAYS

The first time I posted a chicken tenders recipe on Instagram, it went viral, so we made it into a series: All About Chicken Tenders! The idea is that you coat chicken mini fillets in cornflakes, bake or air fry them until crispy and then dip them into a delicious sauce. Below are three of my favourite sauces. These are ideal as a snack or will make a meal if accompanied by chips or wedges.

120g cornflakes

1 tsp salt

1 tsp smoked paprika

1 tsp garlic granules

1 tsp onion granules

1 tsp dried parsley

2 eggs

600g chicken mini fillets

For the creamy peri-peri sauce

½ tbsp extra virgin olive oil

2 cloves of garlic, finely chopped

4 tbsp peri-peri sauce

2 tbsp mascarpone

½ tbsp peri-peri seasoning

1 tsp smoked paprika

½ tbsp red wine vinegar

1–2 tbsp lemon juice

2–3 tbsp boiling water

½ tbsp dried parsley

For the BBQ cajun sauce

2 tbsp BBQ sauce

2 tbsp runny honey

½ tbsp light soy sauce

1 tsp cajun seasoning

½ tsp cayenne pepper

½ tsp smoked paprika

a squeeze of lemon juice

1 plump clove of garlic, peeled and finely chopped

For the chilli sesame sauce

1 tbsp dark soy sauce

3 tbsp sweet chilli sauce

2 tbsp ketchup

3 tbsp runny honey

3 tbsp rice wine vinegar

1–2 cloves of garlic, peeled and finely chopped

1 tbsp sesame seeds

1. Preheat the oven to 190°C (170°C fan/375°F/Gas 5) and line a baking tray with baking paper.

2. Put the cornflakes, salt, smoked paprika, garlic granules, onion granules and dried parsley into a food processor and blitz to a fine crumb, then transfer to a large bowl. Beat the eggs in a medium bowl.

3. Dip each piece of chicken into the egg, then coat in the cornflake mixture and transfer to the prepared baking tray. Bake in the oven for 15–20 minutes. Alternatively, cook in an air fryer at 200°C for 8–10 minutes.

4. To make the creamy peri-peri sauce, heat the oil in a non-stick frying pan over a medium heat and fry the garlic for 1–2 minutes until fragrant, then add the peri-peri sauce and mascarpone. Bring to a low simmer and cook for 2 minutes. Add the peri-peri seasoning, smoked paprika, red wine vinegar and lemon juice, stir to combine and simmer for 3–4 minutes until reduced. Finally, add the boiling water to loosen the sauce and stir in the dried parsley. Allow to cool, then transfer to a sauce pot.

5. To make the BBQ cajun sauce, combine all the ingredients in a small saucepan over a low-medium heat and once the sauce starts to bubble and thicken, remove from the heat. Allow to cool, then transfer to a sauce pot.

6. To make the chilli sesame sauce, combine all the ingredients except the sesame seeds in a small saucepan over a medium heat and simmer for 2 minutes, then add the sesame seeds. Allow to cool, then transfer to a sauce pot.

7. Transfer the tenders to airtight containers and store in the fridge for up to 3 days.

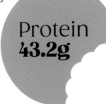

Protein
43.2g

Crispy Sweet Chilli Chicken
WITH STICKY RICE

Get stuck in to the crispiest chicken, tossed in a tangy and sticky sweet chilli sauce. This is a lighter take on the classic takeaway dish of crispy chilli chicken, but it sacrifices no flavour or texture. Best served hot.

2 chicken breasts (400g)
1 tbsp dark soy sauce
1 tsp sesame oil
1 egg white, lightly beaten
90g cornflour
1 tsp groundnut oil
1 clove of garlic, peeled and grated
10g fresh ginger, peeled and grated
1 red pepper, thinly sliced
3–4 spring onions, sliced into 3–4cm pieces
low-calorie cooking spray

For the sweet chilli sauce

1 tbsp dark soy sauce
2 tbsp light soy sauce
1 tbsp sweet chilli sauce
2 tbsp honey

To serve

240g sticky rice
sesame seeds
150g leafy green salad

1. Preheat the oven to 180°C (160°C fan/350°F/Gas 4) and line a baking tray with baking paper.

2. Lay the chicken breasts flat on a board and butterfly them by slicing each one through the middle to create four thinner breasts, then cut into thin strips. Transfer to a large bowl and add the soy sauce, sesame oil and egg white, then mix until combined.

3. Put the cornflour into a separate large bowl. Dip each piece of chicken into the cornflour and toss until coated all over, then transfer to the prepared baking tray or into an air fryer basket. Spray all over with low-calorie cooking spray. Bake in the oven for 20–25 minutes, flipping once or twice during the cooking time. Alternatively, cook in an air fryer at 200°C for 10–12 minutes.

4. Meanwhile, bring a large saucepan of water to the boil and cook the sticky rice according to the packet instructions.

5. In a small bowl, mix together the chilli sauce ingredients.

6. Heat the groundnut oil in a non-stick frying pan over a medium heat and fry the garlic and ginger for 1–2 minutes until fragrant. Add the red pepper and fry for a further 2 minutes, then add the sweet chilli sauce. Allow the sauce to simmer for 30 seconds, then add the crispy chicken pieces. Toss the chicken with the sauce until coated and sticky, then add the spring onion and toss for a minute more.

7. Transfer the rice and chicken to airtight containers and garnish with the sesame seeds. Store in the fridge for up to 4 days. Serve with the leafy green salad.

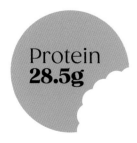

Protein
28.5g

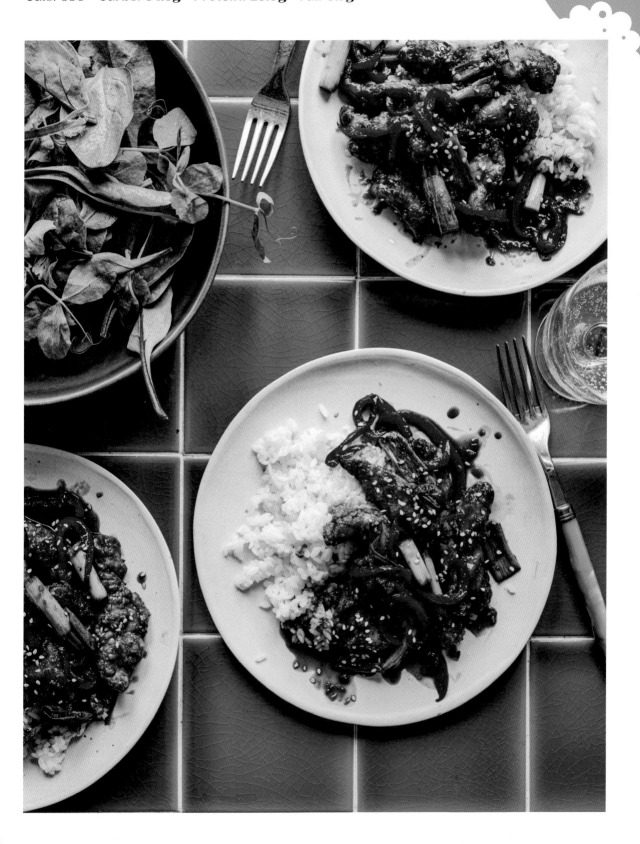

Serves: **4**   Prep time: **5 mins**   Cook time: **25 mins**
Cals: **488**   Carbs: **63.6g**   Protein: **40.3g**   Fat: **9.8g**

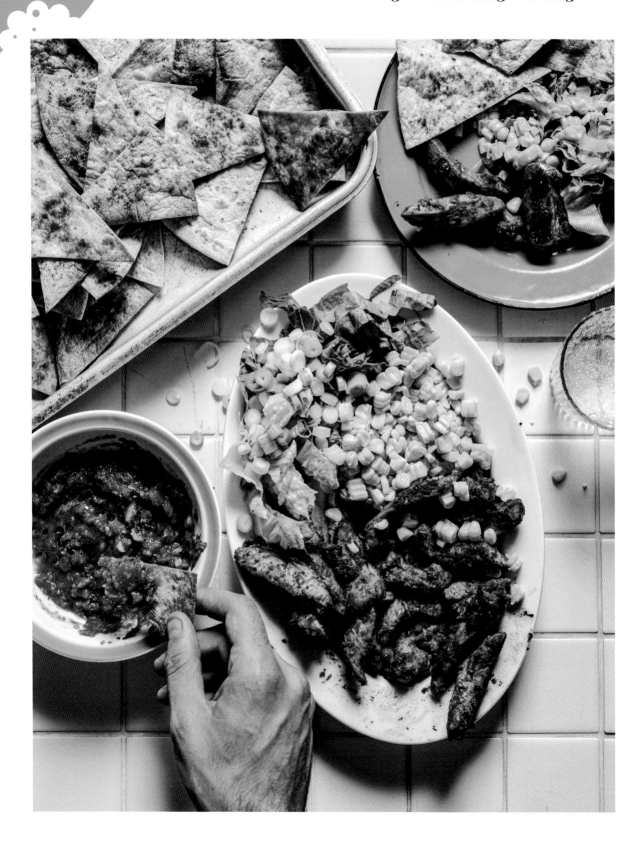

Chipotle Chicken
WITH AIR-FRYER TORTILLA CHIPS & BLENDER SALSA

Crunchy air-fried tortilla chips and juicy chipotle chicken topped off with a punchy, six-ingredient blender salsa makes this a seriously satisfying meal prep recipe – the fact that it's ready in 30 minutes and involves almost no hands-on cooking is just a bonus! This is light in calories and low in fat but sacrifices nothing in the way of flavour or texture. Can be served either hot or cold.

500g chicken breast, sliced
  into thin strips
½ tbsp extra virgin olive oil
1½ tbsp chipotle paste
juice of ½ lime
2 cloves of garlic, peeled
  and crushed
½ tsp salt
low-calorie cooking spray

For the tortilla chips
6 tortilla wraps
2 tsp smoked paprika

For the blender salsa
½ x 400g tin of chopped tomatoes
juice of ½ lime
a small bunch of fresh coriander
1 clove of garlic, peeled
½ onion, roughly chopped
1 fresh jalapeño, deseeded and
  chopped, or 1 tbsp pickled
  jalapeños and brine (optional)

To serve
1 large romaine lettuce, shredded
140g tinned sweetcorn
3 spring onions, finely chopped

1. Combine the chicken, oil, chipotle paste, lime juice, garlic and salt in a large bowl and mix well until the chicken is coated all over, then transfer to an air fryer basket and cook at 200°C for 12–15 minutes, flipping once, until cooked through. Alternatively, heat a few sprays of low-calorie cooking spray in a non-stick frying pan over a medium heat and cook the chicken for 5–10 minutes.

2. Slice the tortillas into eight triangles and transfer to an air fryer basket. Sprinkle over the paprika and spray with cooking spray, then cook at 200°C for 4–6 minutes until crunchy. Alternatively, place on a baking tray lined with baking paper and bake at 180°C (160°C fan/350°F/Gas 4) for 10 minutes.

3. Meanwhile, combine all the salsa ingredients in a blender and blend until combined, then transfer to sauce pots.

4. Divide the chicken among airtight containers, then add the lettuce, sweetcorn and spring onions. Store the tortilla chips in separate containers to keep them crunchy. This will keep in the fridge for up to 4 days.

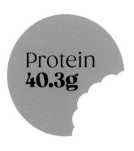

Protein
40.3g

Serves: **4**   Prep time: **15 mins**   Cook time: **35 mins**

Cals: **443**   Carbs: **37.6g**   Protein: **52.5g**   Fat: **10.1g**

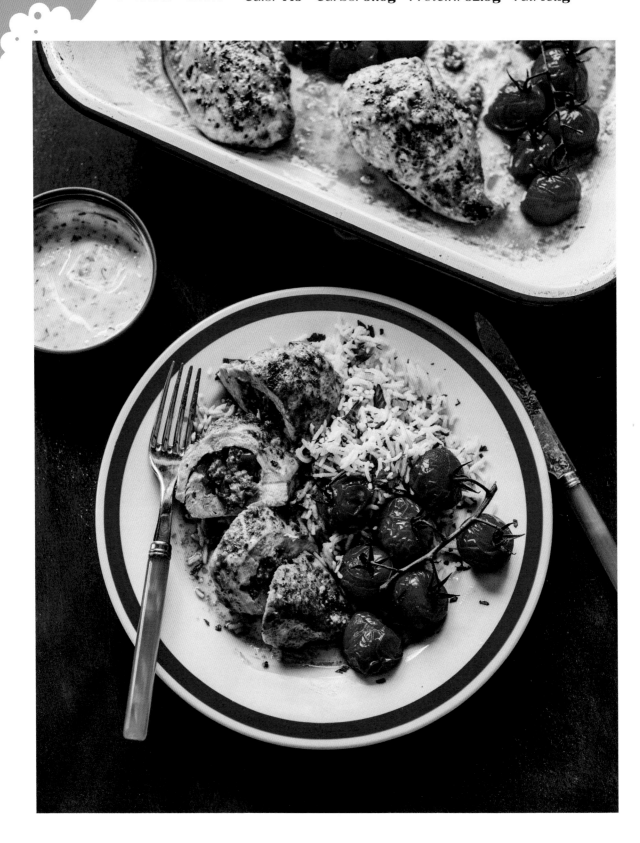

Chorizo-stuffed Chicken Breasts
WITH ROASTED VINE TOMATOES, LIME & CORIANDER RICE & GARLIC & HERB DIP

This recipe is just a few really simple components chucked together to make the perfect lunchbox. Juicy and cheesy chorizo-stuffed chicken breasts (which taste out of this world!), jammy roasted cherry tomatoes, zesty rice and a creamy garlic and herb dip, all ready in 25 minutes and packed to the brim with flavour!

4 medium chicken breasts
2 tbsp light cream cheese
12 chorizo slices
1 small sweet Romano pepper, finely chopped
20g reduced-fat Cheddar cheese, finely grated
1 tbsp Cajun seasoning
250g vine cherry tomatoes
500g cooked basmati rice, cooled, or 165g uncooked basmati rice, cooked
juice of 2 limes
30g fresh coriander, finely chopped
low-calorie cooking spray
salt and freshly ground black pepper

For the garlic and herb dip
150g fat-free yoghurt
juice of ½ lime
1 tsp garlic granules
1 tsp dried parsley

1. Preheat the oven to 190°C (170°C fan/375°F/Gas 5).

2. Slice open the chicken breasts lengthways, then stuff with the cream cheese, chorizo slices (folded over), Romano pepper and Cheddar. Close the chicken breasts (you can use toothpicks if you like, but it's not essential), then coat with the Cajun seasoning and spray with low-calorie cooking spray. Place in a baking dish and bake in the oven for 25 minutes, or until cooked through. Alternatively, cook in an air fryer at 200°C for 15–20 minutes.

3. Put the tomatoes into a small baking dish and bake in the oven for 6–8 minutes until nearly bursting. Alternatively, cook in an air fryer at 180°C for 6 minutes.

4. Meanwhile, put the rice into a large bowl and add the lime juice and coriander, reserving a little coriander for the dip. Season lightly, then mix until combined.

5. Combine all the ingredients for the dip in a separate bowl, add the reserved coriander and stir well, then transfer to sauce pots.

6. Transfer the chicken, rice and tomatoes to airtight containers and store in the fridge for up to 3 days.

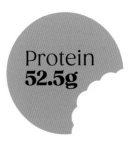

Protein
52.5g

Air-fried Chimichurri Steak Bites
WITH TOMATO COUSCOUS

Succulent and garlicky air-fried steak bites are tossed in a punchy and vibrant chimichurri sauce. This is a lower calorie and high-protein lunchtime option that is filled to the brim with flavour.

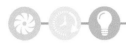

2 sirloin steaks (400g), diced
1 tbsp light soy sauce
½ tsp onion granules
½ tsp garlic granules
salt and freshly ground
   black pepper

For the chimichurri

15g unsalted butter
3 cloves of garlic, peeled
   and crushed
1 shallot, peeled and finely
   chopped
a small bunch of fresh parsley,
   very finely chopped
a small bunch of fresh coriander,
   very finely chopped
1 tbsp extra virgin olive oil
1 tsp dried oregano
1 tbsp red wine vinegar
a pinch of chilli flakes
juice of 1 lime
a pinch of salt

For the garlic sauce

100g fat-free natural yoghurt
1–2 cloves of garlic, peeled and
   finely grated
juice of 1 lemon

To serve

2 x 110g packets of flavoured
   couscous (any flavour of
   your choice)
4 medium tomatoes, chopped

1. First, cook the couscous according to the packet instructions, then set aside.

2. In a bowl, whisk together the garlic sauce ingredients and transfer to sauce pots.

3. Put the steak into a separate bowl, add the soy sauce, onion granules, garlic granules and some salt and pepper and stir to coat. Transfer to an air fryer and cook at 200°C for 7 minutes. Alternatively, cook in a non-stick frying pan for 5–7 minutes.

4. Next, make the chimichurri. Melt the butter in a frying pan over a medium heat and fry the garlic and shallot for 2 minutes, then add the parsley, coriander, olive oil, oregano, red wine vinegar, chilli flakes, lime juice, salt and 1½ tablespoons water. Cook for 2–3 minutes, stirring regularly, until reduced, then add the steak bites. Toss well until coated, then remove from the heat.

5. Just before serving, stir the tomatoes into the couscous.

6. Transfer the couscous and steak bites to airtight containers and drizzle over any remaining chimichurri sauce from the pan. Store in the fridge for up to 4 days.

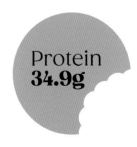

Protein
34.9g

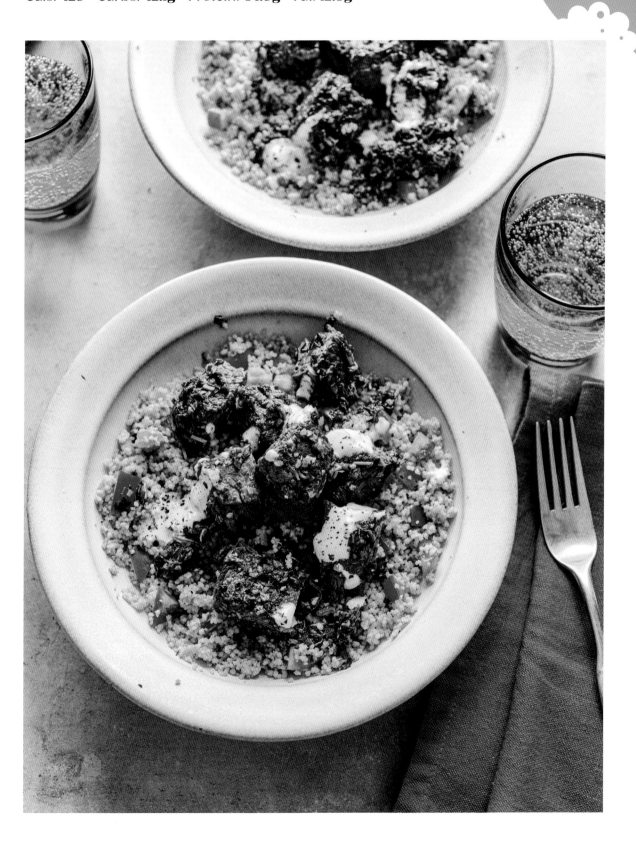

Harissa Roast Chicken
& CHIPS

I was unsure whether to put this recipe in the book because, at first, it might not strike you as a typical 'meal prep' dish. But when I cooked it for my wife, Megan, and her mum, they absolutely loved it and told me it had to go in the book. It was such a satisfying meal, full of amazing flavours, and it actually turned out to be very suitable for meal prep, yielding two delicious breasts and two legs, plus the chips and gravy as sides. I love the air-frying technique as well, as it saves so much time. Just be careful it's cooked through before carving because different air fryers will cook at slightly differently rates.

75g rose harissa paste
4 cloves of garlic, peeled
   and crushed
1 medium chicken
½ lemon
½ orange
1 tbsp extra virgin olive oil
salt and freshly ground
   black pepper

For the chips
1kg Maris Piper potatoes, cut into
   equal-sized chips
1 tbsp extra-virgin olive oil

For the harissa gravy
1 chicken stock cube, mixed with
   200ml boiling water
½ tbsp cornflour, mixed with a
   splash of cold water

1. Preheat the oven to 180°C (160°C fan/350°F/Gas 4).

2. Mix together the rose harissa paste and garlic in a small bowl. Stuff the cavity of the chicken with the lemon and orange, drizzle the olive oil all over the chicken and season generously all over with salt and pepper.

For oven cooking:
3. Transfer the chicken to a baking tray, cover tightly with tin foil and roast in the oven for 1 hour 40 minutes, basting and smothering the chicken with the rose harissa mixture halfway through.

4. Put the potatoes into a baking tray, toss with the oil and cook in the oven for 35-45 minutes, tossing a few times.

For air frying:
5. Place the chicken, breast side down, in an air fryer and cook at 190°C for 30 minutes. Collect the juices from the bottom of the air fryer, then flip the chicken over and drizzle over the juices and the rose harissa mixture. Tightly cover with tin foil and place back in the air fryer for a further 25 minutes.

6. If you have a dual air fryer, then you can cook the chips at the same time as the roast chicken.

7. If not, then remove the chicken from the air fryer and clean out the basket, then add the potatoes. Toss with the oil and season with salt, then cook in the air fryer at 200°C for 30 minutes, tossing a few times.

8. To make the harissa gravy, transfer the roasting juices to a saucepan and add the chicken stock and cornflour. Simmer for 3–4 minutes until thickened, then transfer to sauce pots.

9. Carve the chicken into breasts and legs and transfer to airtight containers with the chips and gravy pots. Keep in the fridge for 3–4 days.

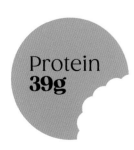

Protein
39g

Serves: 4   Prep time: **5 mins**   Cook time: **1 hr 40 mins**
Cals: **565**   Carbs: **52.2g**   Protein: **39g**   Fat: **23.9g**

139

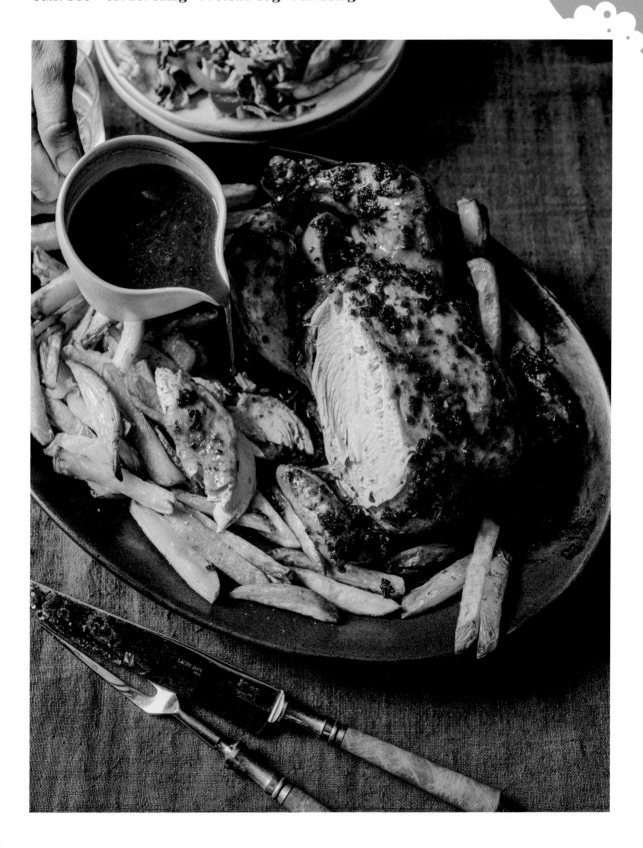

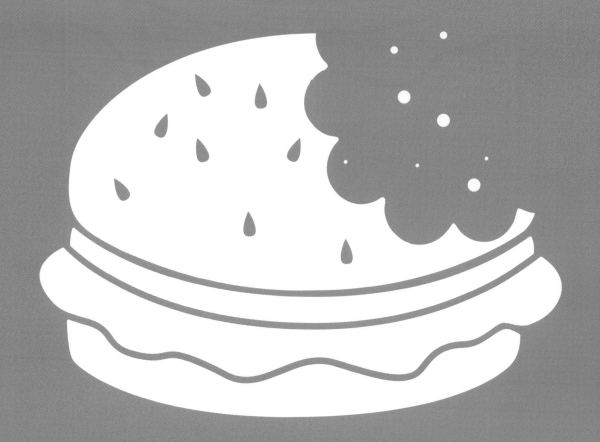

Favourite
Fakeaways

Sticky Korean Popcorn Chicken Rice Bowl

This might be the freshest and most moreish meal prep recipe you could ever make! Crispy popcorn chicken tossed in a sticky and spicy Korean sauce, served with quick-pickled cucumber slices – so good. This healthy and high-protein packed lunch recipe will make you feel like you've just visited your favourite street food market.

2 egg whites
1 tbsp light soy sauce
500g chicken breast, diced
75g cornflour
1 tbsp groundnut oil

For the quick-pickled cucumbers

1 cucumber, thinly sliced
2 tbsp rice wine vinegar
2 tsp granulated sugar

For the sticky Korean sauce

1 tbsp gochujang (Korean chilli paste)
1½ tbsp light soy sauce
3 tbsp runny honey
1 tbsp rice wine vinegar

To serve

240g jasmine rice
80g watercress salad
2 spring onions, thinly sliced
sesame seeds
sriracha mayonnaise

1. Preheat the oven to 190°C (170°C fan/375°F/Gas 5).

2. First, make the quick-pickled cucumbers. Put the cucumber, vinegar and sugar into a large bowl and mix to combine. Set aside while you prepare everything else.

3. Next, make the chicken. In a separate large bowl, whisk together the egg whites and soy sauce, then add the chicken and stir to coat. Pour the cornflour onto a large baking tray, add the chicken and toss to coat. Transfer to a separate baking tray and drizzle over the groundnut oil or divide the chicken pieces between two air fryer baskets and add ½ tablespoon of oil per basket. Bake in the oven for 20–25 minutes until crispy or cook in an air fryer at 190°C for 15 minutes, flipping the chicken halfway through.

4. Meanwhile, bring a large saucepan of water to the boil and cook the rice according to the packet instructions, then drain.

5. Combine the sticky Korean sauce ingredients in a small saucepan and cook over a medium heat for 2–4 minutes until bubbling, then pour into a large bowl. Add the crispy chicken and toss to coat.

6. Transfer to airtight containers with the rice and watercress salad. Garnish with the spring onions, sesame seeds and sriracha mayonnaise. Store the pickled cucumbers in a separate airtight container. This will keep in the fridge for up to 3 days.

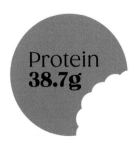

Protein
38.7g

Serves: **4**   Prep time: **10 mins**   Cook time: **25 mins**

Cals: **591**   Carbs: **88.8g**   Protein: **38.7g**   Fat: **10.9g**

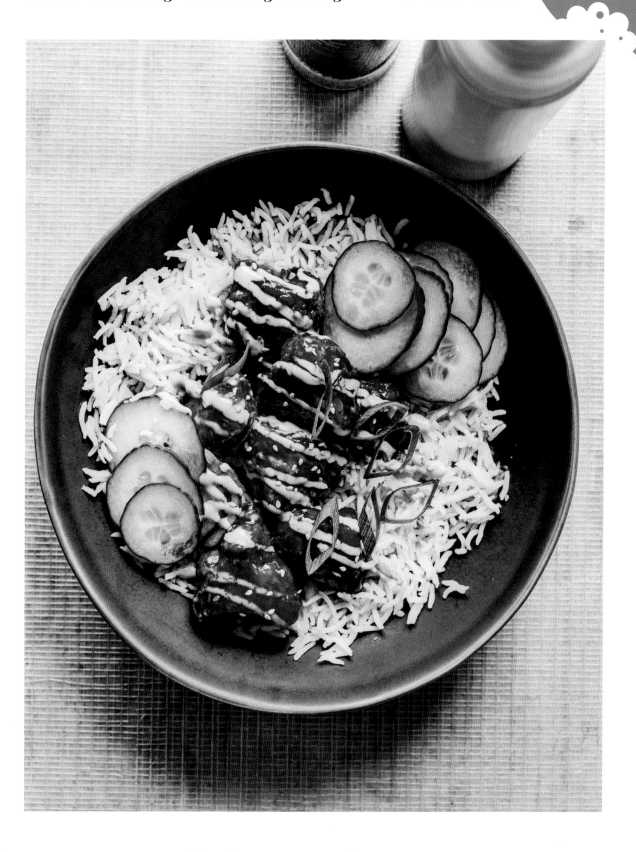

Chicken Katsu Curry

In this recipe, I've successfully turned one of the nation's favourite dishes into a healthier packed lunch option, featuring chicken coated in panko breadcrumbs and shallow-fried until wonderfully golden and crispy, teamed with a super-easy, make-ahead katsu curry sauce. This is lighter than any takeaway you'll get delivered to your doorstep but just as tasty.

For the crispy chicken

2 large chicken breasts
2 egg whites
2 tbsp plain flour
100g panko breadcrumbs
2 tbsp groundnut oil
salt and freshly ground
   black pepper

For the katsu curry sauce

75g katsu curry paste (available at
   most supermarkets)
120ml reduced-fat coconut milk
1 tbsp tahini
1 tsp runny honey
1 tbsp light soy sauce
½ tsp mild chilli powder
juice of ½ lime

To serve

240g basmati rice
1 cucumber, sliced
1–2 carrots, cut into matchsticks
2 spring onions, sliced
sesame seeds

1. Preheat the oven to 180°C (160°C fan/350°F/Gas 4) and line a baking tray with baking paper.

2. Lay the chicken breasts flat on a board and butterfly them by slicing each one through the middle to create four thinner breasts. Put the egg into a bowl and put the flour and panko breadcrumbs onto two separate plates before lightly seasoning both with salt and pepper. Coat the chicken breasts in the flour, then dip in the beaten egg and finally coat in the breadcrumbs. Press the breadcrumbs into the chicken breasts to ensure they are coated all over.

3. Heat the oil in a large frying pan over a medium heat and cook the chicken for 3–4 minutes on each side until browned. Transfer the chicken to the prepared baking tray and bake for 15–20 minutes until crispy. Alternatively, cook in an air fryer at 200°C for 12–15 minutes.

4. Meanwhile, bring a large saucepan of water to the boil and cook the rice according to the packet instructions, then drain.

5. In a large bowl or jug, whisk together the katsu curry sauce ingredients until combined, then transfer to four sauce pots.

6. Divide the rice and chicken among airtight containers and top with the cucumber, carrots, spring onions and sesame seeds. Store in the refrigerator for up to 4 days.

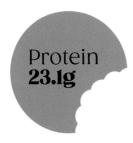

Protein
23.1g

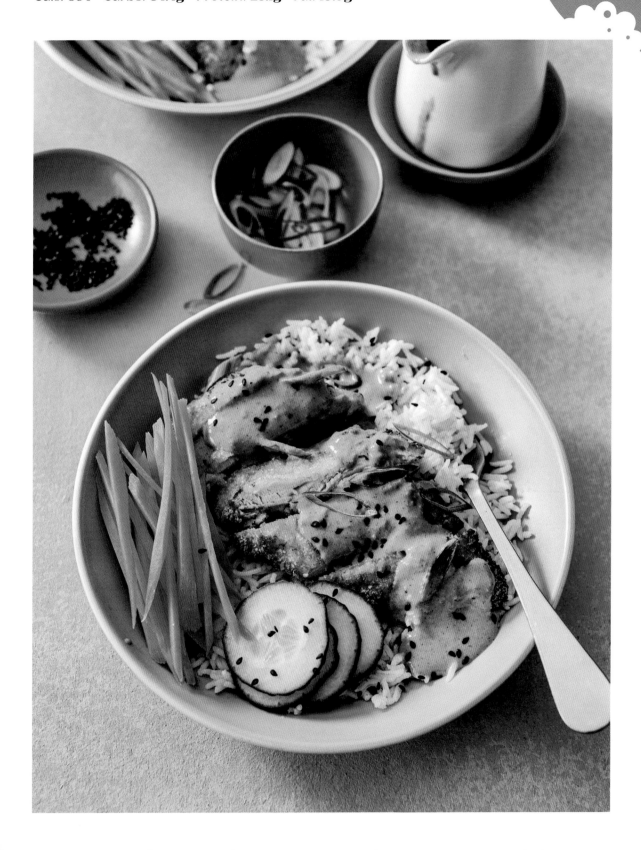

Serves: **4**   Prep time: **5 mins, plus marinating**
Cook time: **50 mins**
Cals: **385**   Carbs: **26.9g**   Protein: **41.4g**   Fat: **12.8g**

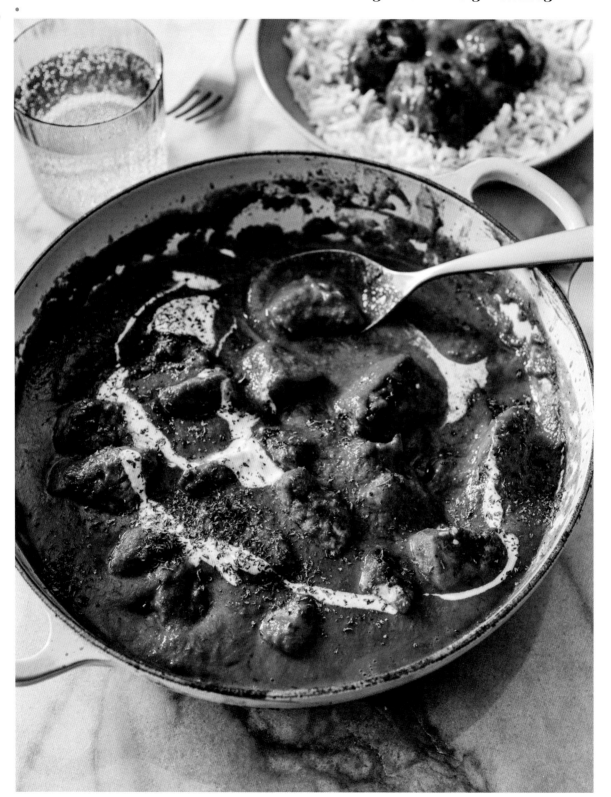

Butter Chicken Curry

This is the ultimate butter chicken fakeaway. I've managed to keep the calories low while still using real butter, which gives it a wonderfully rich flavour. It works perfectly as a light but flavoursome meal prep option as it is, but to bulk it out, add half a naan per portion. Best served hot.

500g chicken breast, diced
1 tbsp groundnut oil
20g unsalted butter
1 onion, diced
3 cloves of garlic, peeled
  and grated
20g fresh ginger, peeled
  and grated
1 tsp ground cumin
1 tsp ground coriander
½ tsp ground turmeric
½ tsp smoked paprika
1 x 400g tin of chopped tomatoes
250ml chicken stock
150ml light coconut milk

For the marinade
1 tsp ground cumin
1 tsp ground turmeric
1 tsp mild chilli powder
1 tsp paprika
1 tsp garam masala
1 clove of garlic, peeled
  and grated
10g fresh ginger, peeled
  and grated
3 tbsp fat-free natural yoghurt

To serve
240g basmati rice
a pinch of dried fenugreek
  or parsley
100g fat-free natural yoghurt

1. Combine all the marinade ingredients in a large bowl and add the chicken, then mix well until the chicken is fully coated. Cover and set aside in the fridge to marinate for 4–6 hours if you have time, but if you're in a rush then don't worry about it!

2. Bring a large saucepan of water to the boil and cook the rice according to the packet instructions, then drain.

3. Heat the oil in a large, non-stick saucepan over a medium heat and cook the chicken for 10 minutes, flipping once or twice, until cooked through. Remove from the pan and set aside.

4. Melt the butter in the same pan, then add the onion and fry gently over a low heat for 5–10 minutes until deeply golden. Add the garlic and ginger and fry for 1–2 minutes before adding the cumin, coriander, turmeric and smoked paprika. Toast the spices for 1 minute, then add the chopped tomatoes and chicken stock. Bring to a simmer and cook for 15 minutes until the sauce has reduced and thickened.

5. Once reduced, transfer the sauce to a blender and blend until smooth. Transfer the sauce back to the pan and add the chicken and coconut milk. Stir to combine, then bring to a low simmer and cook for 5 minutes, or until it has reached your desired consistency.

6. Transfer the rice and butter chicken to airtight containers and garnish with the dried fenugreek or parsley. Divide the yoghurt among sauce pots to serve with the curry. This will keep in the fridge for up to 4 days.

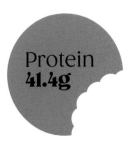

Protein
41.4g

Serves: **4**   Prep time: **10 mins**   Cook time: **1 hr**
Cals: **750**   Carbs: **72.4g**   Protein: **51.3g**   Fat: **29.9g**

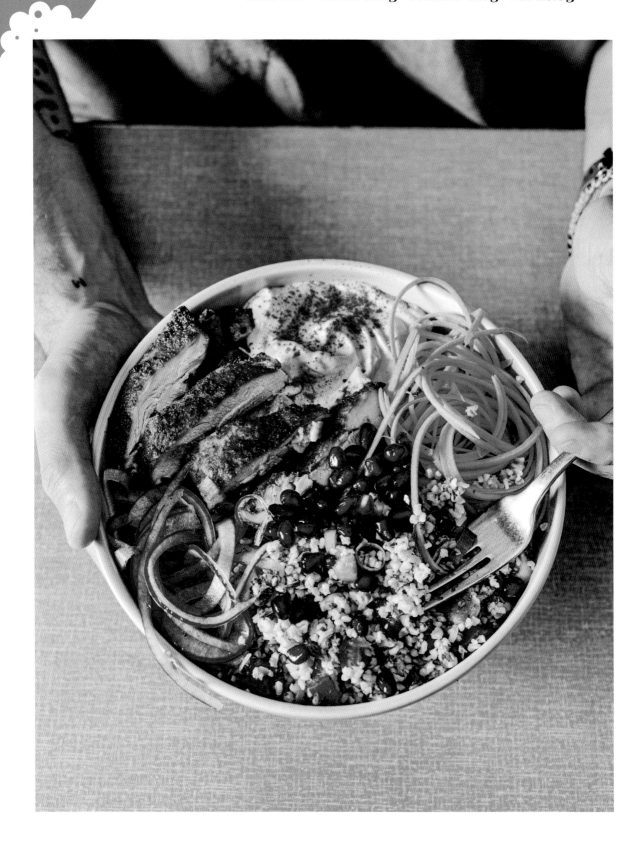

Chicken Shawarma Naked Bowl

This Middle Eastern-inspired shawarma bowl is out of this world. The deep, bold flavours of the chicken will warm you from the inside out. I've paired it with a quick, easy and super-fresh tabbouleh. The chicken can be served hot or cold.

1 tsp ground cumin
1 tsp ground turmeric
1 tsp ground coriander
½ tsp ground cinnamon
1 tsp mild chilli powder
1 tsp garlic granules
1 tsp paprika
½ tsp cloves (optional)
½ tsp salt
600g skinless, boneless
  chicken thighs
1 tbsp extra virgin olive oil
2 tbsp fat-free Greek yoghurt

For the tabbouleh
250g bulgur wheat
500ml hot vegetable stock
½ tsp salt, plus extra to taste
2 tbsp extra virgin olive oil
zest and juice of 2 lemons
6–8 tomatoes, diced
2 spring onions, thinly sliced
2 bunches of fresh curly parsley,
  finely chopped
freshly ground black pepper

To serve
1 carrot, peeled and julienned
4 tbsp pickled red onions
240g hummus per portion
100g pomegranate seeds
2 pitta breads, halved (optional
  and not included in calories)

1. First, cook the bulgur wheat for the tabbouleh. Put the bulgur wheat into a large, heatproof bowl and pour over the hot vegetable stock. Add the salt, stir to combine, then cover and leave to absorb the liquid for 30–60 minutes.

2. Preheat the oven to 180°C (160°C fan/350°F/Gas 4).

3. Put all the spices and the salt for the chicken into a large bowl and stir to combine. Coat the chicken thighs in the olive oil, then add to the bowl with spices along with the Greek yoghurt. Mix well until the chicken is coated all over.

4. Transfer the chicken to a large baking dish or loaf tin and bake for 35 minutes. Alternatively, cook in an air fryer at 190°C for 15–20 minutes.

5. In a small bowl, mix together the olive oil and lemon juice for the tabbouleh, then pour into the bulgur wheat and mix together. Add the lemon zest, tomatoes, spring onions and parsley and mix well until combined. Season to taste.

6. Divide the tabbouleh among airtight containers, then slice the chicken thighs and add to the tabbouleh along with the carrots, pickled onions, hummus, pomegranate seeds and pitta bread, if using. This will keep for up to 4 days.

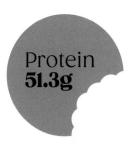

Protein
51.3g

Massaman Chicken Curry
WITH FRAGRANT LIME BASMATI RICE

A vibrant Thai curry served with delicious, sticky and fragrant jasmine rice. This is a very simple recipe to follow, and you can easily chuck in any other crunchy veg you might fancy. The curry will get thicker the longer you simmer it – I would aim for at least a medium thickness so the sauce doesn't run into the rice when boxing up for meal prep.

1 tbsp groundnut oil
2 shallots, peeled and finely chopped
2 cloves of garlic, peeled and grated
20g fresh ginger, peeled and grated
4 tbsp massaman curry paste
1 x 400ml tin of reduced-fat coconut milk
300ml boiling water
1 tbsp fish sauce
2 tbsp finely chopped fresh coriander
1 tbsp runny honey
juice of ½ lime
1 tbsp smooth peanut butter
½–1 tbsp sriracha (or to taste; optional)
500g chicken breast, very thinly sliced
300g waxy potatoes, cut into medium-sized chunks

To serve
180g uncooked jasmine rice
2 lime leaves, torn in half
30 unsalted peanuts, toasted and chopped
1 pak choi, thinly sliced
fresh coriander, leaves picked
4 lime wedges

1. Heat the oil in a large, deep saucepan over a high heat and fry the shallots, garlic and ginger for 2 minutes, stirring regularly, then add the curry paste. Cook out the curry paste for 1–2 minutes until thickened, then add the coconut milk and boiling water. Bring to a rapid simmer, then add the fish sauce, coriander, honey, lime juice, peanut butter and sriracha, if using, and stir to combine.

2. Add the chicken and cook for 5–10 minutes until the edges have sealed and you can see no more pink. Add the potatoes and cook for 15–20 minutes until fork-tender. Continue to simmer for a further 5–10 minutes until the curry has reached your desired consistency.

3. Meanwhile, bring a large saucepan of water to the boil, add the lime leaves and rice and cook according to the packet instructions, then drain.

4. Divide the rice among airtight containers, packing it to one side, then pour the curry into the other half, keeping them separate. Garnish with the peanuts, pak choi, coriander and lime wedges. Store in the fridge for 3–4 days.

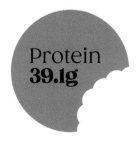

Protein
39.1g

Serves: **4**   Prep time: **5 mins**   Cook time: **1 hr 5 mins**
Cals: **572**   Carbs: **63.7g**   Protein: **39.1g**   Fat: **19.4g**

151

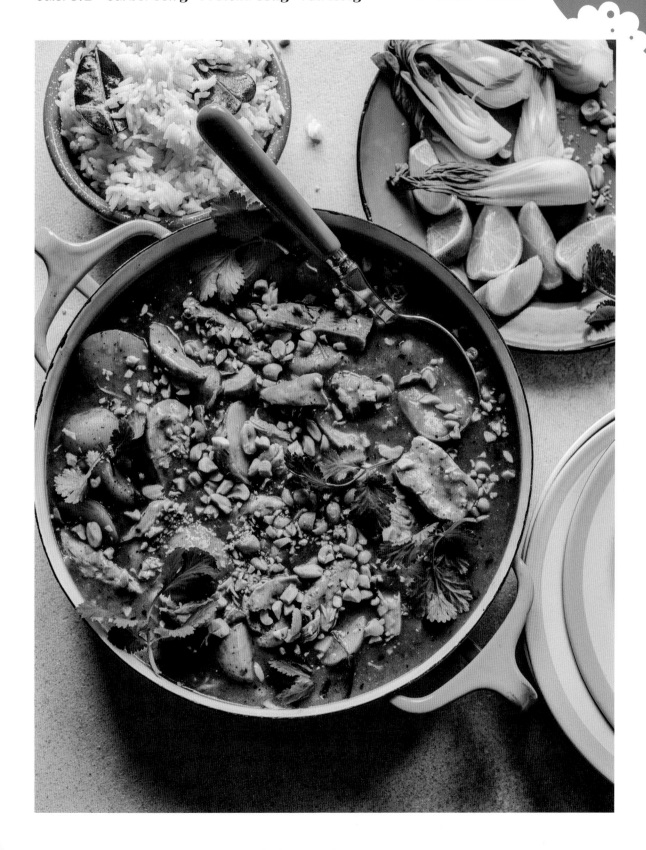

Fish Fillet Burgers

This is inspired by everyone's favourite fish burger from that fast food restaurant with the golden arches … except this is way more filling, fresh, tasty and packed with more high-quality protein. Breaded cod fillets, air fried or baked until crispy, are packed between two toasted brioche buns with a simple homemade tartar sauce and cheese. Best served hot.

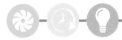

50g golden breadcrumbs
½ tsp smoked paprika
1 egg, beaten
2 tbsp plain flour
4 x 120g cod fillets
4 brioche buns
4 American cheese slices
low-calorie cooking spray
salt and freshly ground
  black pepper

For the tartar sauce

1 tbsp light mayonnaise
3 tbsp fat-free Greek yoghurt
1 tbsp lemon juice
½ tbsp dill, finely chopped
1 tbsp capers, drained
  and chopped
½ tbsp caper brine
1 tsp Dijon mustard
½ tsp freshly ground black pepper

1. Preheat the oven to 220°C (200°C fan/425°F/Gas 7) and line a baking tray with baking paper.

2. In a large bowl, mix the breadcrumbs with the smoked paprika and plenty of salt and pepper. Put the egg into a separate bowl and pour the flour onto a large plate.

3. Pat the cod fillets dry with kitchen paper, then season with salt and pepper. If your cod fillets are too long and thin to make nice, square patties, fold them in half. Dip the cod into the flour to coat all over, then dip in the beaten egg and then in the breadcrumbs, making sure the fillets are well covered. Spray with low-calorie cooking spray, then transfer to the prepared baking tray and bake in the oven for 15 minutes, flipping once. Alternatively, cook in an air fryer at 200°C for 12 minutes until crispy.

4. Meanwhile, mix together all the ingredients for the tartar sauce in a small bowl.

5. Slice and lightly toast the buns, then add a cheese slice and crispy fish fillet to each bottom bun. Spread the tartar sauce onto the top buns and place on top.

6. Tightly wrap in cling film or transfer to airtight containers and refrigerate for up to 3 days.

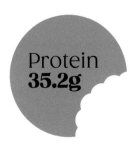

Protein
35.2g

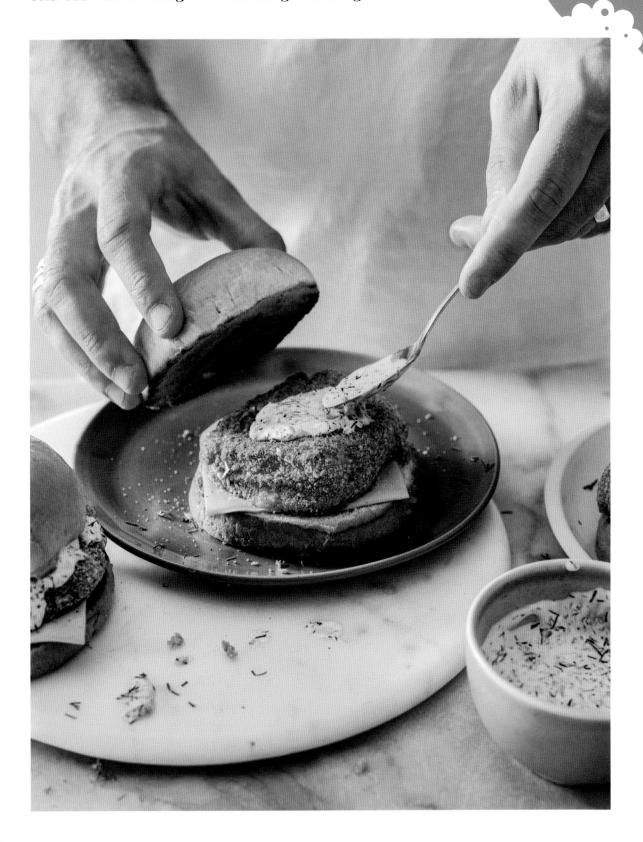

9 780241 693964

Serves: **4**   Prep time: **10 mins**   Cook time: **15 mins**
Cals: **495**   Carbs: **29.3g**   Protein: **49.3g**   Fat: **19.3g**

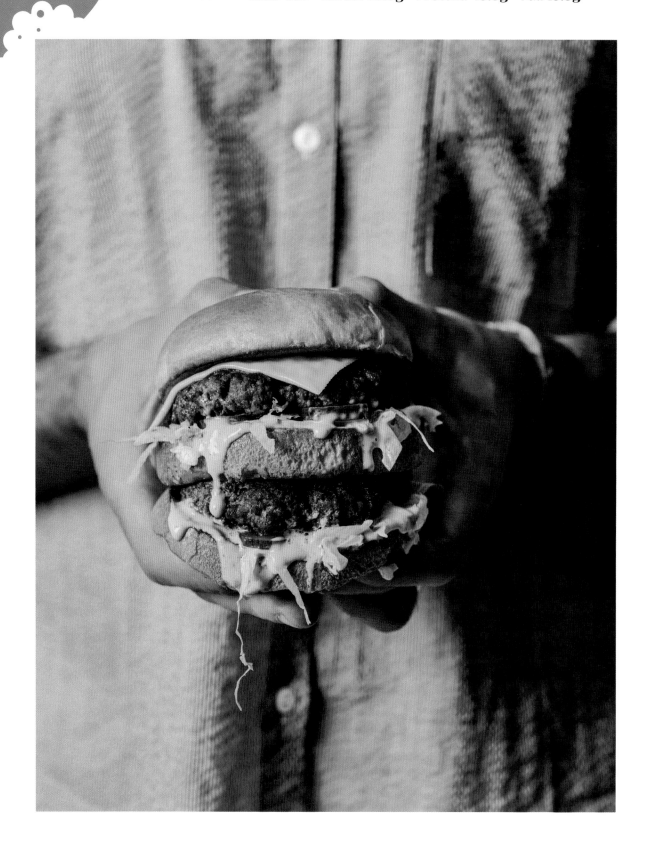

Ultimate Double-stacked Beef Burger

Treat yourself for lunch with my ultimate fakeaway burger! These are wholesome, hearty and super high in protein, as well as being really easy to make and even tastier (and more satisfying) than a takeaway. I've whipped together a lighter burger sauce, which saves on calories but still has that distinctive flavour that we all know and love.

800g lean minced beef (5% fat)
4 American cheese slices
6 brioche burger buns, sliced and toasted
a large handful of thinly sliced iceberg lettuce
½ onion, finely chopped
50g pickled sliced gherkins
low-calorie cooking spray
salt and freshly ground black pepper

For the burger sauce
3 tbsp light mayonnaise
3 tbsp reduced-sugar ketchup
1 tbsp yellow mustard
2 tbsp pickle brine
1 tsp garlic granules

1. Mix together the ingredients for the burger sauce in a bowl, then set aside.

2. Divide the beef into eight equal-sized pieces and form into patties, then flatten to roughly 2–3cm thick and season with salt and black pepper.

3. Heat a few sprays of low-calorie cooking spray in a large, non-stick frying pan and add half the patties. Cook for 3 minutes on each side, then remove from the pan. Repeat with the remaining patties, but this time top the cooked patties with the cheese slices and allow to melt before removing from the pan.

4. Spread four bottom buns with the burger sauce, then top with lettuce, onion, gherkin slices and the beef patties without cheese.

5. Top with 4 bun halves to form the middle buns, then top with more burger sauce, lettuce, gherkin slices and the beef patties with cheese, then close with the top bun.

6. These will keep in the fridge for up to 4 days.

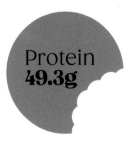

Protein
49.3g

Black Dhal

The hero ingredient in this recipe are the lentils. They are a high-protein superfood and they make this amazing dhal one of the healthiest recipes in the entire book. It's a classic Indian dish that is super comforting thanks to its gentle blend of spices and soup-like consistency. I've used full-fat butter, although less than is used in an authentically cooked black dhal, because it's supposed to be buttery. It is accompanied perfectly by warm naan, which you can use to scoop up the delicious black lentils. Best served hot.

40g unsalted butter

1 onion, chopped

5 cloves of garlic, peeled and finely grated

15g fresh ginger, finely grated

1 tbsp curry powder

½ tsp mild chilli powder or deggi mirch

1 cinnamon stick

2 bay leaves

2 large or 4 medium tomatoes, diced

50g tomato purée

1 tsp salt

2 x 250g packs of cooked beluga lentils

1 tsp garam masala

½ tbsp runny honey

50ml single cream, plus extra to serve

a handful of fresh coriander, to garnish

salt and freshly ground black pepper

2 naans, halved, to serve

fresh coriander, to serve

1. Melt the butter in a large saucepan over a medium heat and add the onion and a pinch of salt. Cook for 8–10 minutes, stirring regularly, until softened and brown. Add the garlic and ginger and cook for a further 3–4 minutes until fragrant.

2. Add the curry powder, chilli powder, cinnamon stick and bay leaves and stir to coat the onion mixture in the spices. Fry over a high heat for 1 minute, then add the tomatoes, tomato purée, a pinch of salt and a splash of water. Cook over a medium heat for 5 minutes.

3. Add 400ml water and 6 tablespoons of the lentils (we add some of the lentils here to add flavour and thickness to the sauce when we eventually blend it). Bring to a low simmer and cook for 20–30 minutes, until the tomatoes have completely broken down.

4. Discard the cinnamon stick and bay leaves, then transfer the sauce to a blender and blend until smooth. Pour back into the pan (you can swill some water in the blender to ensure no sauce is left behind) and add the remaining lentils, garam masala, honey and about 100ml of water (use more or less for a thicker or soupier consistency, it's up to you!). Simmer for 5–10 minutes, then stir in the cream and season to taste.

5. Transfer to airtight containers and store in the fridge for up to 4 days. Drizzle with cream and garnish with fresh coriander before serving with the naans.

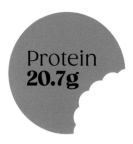

Protein
20.7g

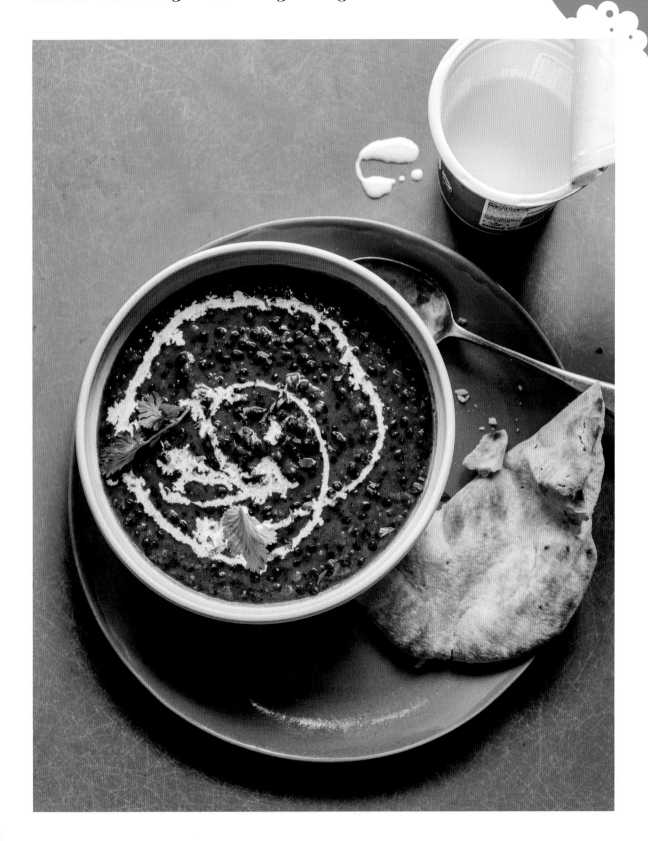

Roasting Tin Fajitas
WITH LIME & CORIANDER SAUCE

I've roasted these fajitas in a tin primarily for ease, but this method also happens to maximize their flavour! Just coat the chicken and veg in the spices, roast them in the oven and the results are wonderful – succulent chicken breast and tender onions and peppers, dripping with juices and full of flavour. Pile it into a wrap for a perfect on-the-go lunch that can be enjoyed hot or cold – all accompanied by a delicious creamy lime and coriander sauce.

4 medium chicken breasts
2 white or red onions, sliced
3 peppers (any colour), sliced
2 tbsp extra virgin olive oil
60g reduced-fat Cheddar cheese, grated
4 tortilla wraps

For the fajita seasoning (or use shop-bought)

1 tbsp ground cumin
1 tbsp smoked paprika
1 tbsp mild chilli powder
½ tbsp garlic granules
½ tbsp onion granules
1 tsp salt

For the lime and coriander sauce

2 tbsp soured cream
100g fat-free Greek yoghurt
a small bunch of fresh coriander
juice of ½ lime
a pinch of salt

1. Preheat the oven to 190°C (170°C fan/375°F/Gas 5) and line a roasting tin or baking tray with baking paper.

2. First, mix together all the ingredients for the fajita seasoning – for best results, grind in a pestle and mortar, otherwise stir together in a bowl.

3. Place the chicken on a board, cover with cling film and use a rolling pin to flatten it to a 2.5cm thickness. Transfer to the prepared roasting tin and add the onions and peppers. Sprinkle over the fajita seasoning and toss to coat, then drizzle with the oil. Bake in the oven for 20 minutes, flipping once, until cooked through. Remove from the oven and slice the chicken breast. Alternatively, cook in an air fryer at 200°C for 15–20 minutes.

4. Meanwhile, put all the lime and coriander sauce ingredients into a blender and blend until smooth, then transfer to sauce pots.

5. Build the fajitas with the chicken and peppers, Cheddar and tortilla wraps. Tightly wrap in cling film or tin foil and store in the fridge for up to 4 days. Add the lime and coriander sauce to the fajita wraps or use it as a dip.

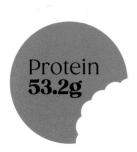

Protein
53.2g

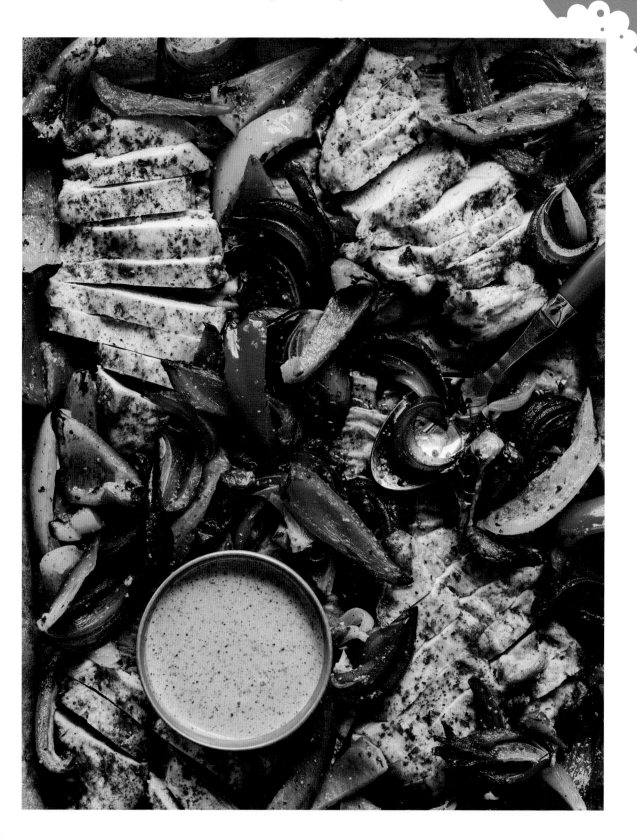

9 780241 693995

Serves: **4**   Prep time: **10 mins**   Cook time: **20 mins**
Cals: **562**   Carbs: **75.4g**   Protein: **25.5g**   Fat: **18.9g**

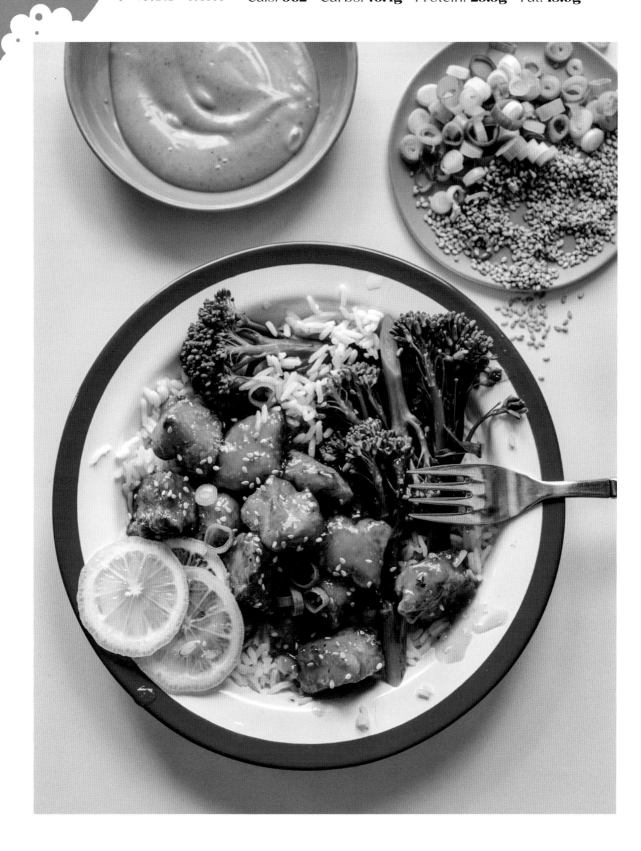

Lemon Pepper Tofu

The flavour of the sauce that coats the crispy tofu pieces in this recipe is super intense and will leave your tastebuds tingling. Tofu is my favourite high-protein non-meat alternative and this recipe is 100 per cent plant-based. This recipe is best served hot.

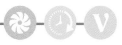

¼ tsp salt
¾ tbsp freshly ground
  black pepper
zest of 3 lemons
60g cornflour, mixed with
  cold water
1 x 450g block of firm tofu, torn
  in to 2–3cm pieces
2 tbsp light soy sauce
1 tbsp groundnut oil, for cooking

For the sticky lemon sauce

zest of 1 lemon
juice of 3 lemons
3 tbsp maple syrup
½ tbsp light soy sauce
1 tsp cornflour mixed with 2 tsp
  of cold water

To serve

240g jasmine or basmati rice
150g Tenderstem broccoli
4 lemon slices
2 spring onions, finely chopped,
sesame seeds
2 tbsp sriracha mayonnaise

1. Preheat the oven to 180°C (160°C fan/350°F/Gas 4) and line a baking tray with baking paper.

2. In a pestle and mortar, grind together the salt, pepper and lemon zest, then transfer to a large bowl with the cornflour and mix until combined. Put the tofu and soy sauce into a separate large bowl and mix until coated, then dip the wet tofu into the cornflour mixture in batches of four to five pieces at a time, ensuring the tofu is coated all over in the cornflour mixture. Transfer to the prepared baking tray.

3. Drizzle the tofu with groundnut oil and toss to coat, then bake in the oven for 15–20 minutes until golden and crisp. Alternatively, cook in an air fryer at 180°C for 8–10 minutes.

4. Meanwhile, bring a large saucepan of water to the boil and cook the rice according to the packet instructions, then drain.

5. Bring a separate saucepan of water to the boil and boil or steam the broccoli until cooked but still crunchy.

6. Combine all the ingredients for the sticky lemon sauce in a saucepan, then bring to a simmer over a medium heat and cook for 3–4 minutes until thick and bubbling. Add the baked tofu and toss to coat.

7. Transfer the rice, tofu, broccoli and lemon slices to airtight containers, then garnish with the spring onions and sesame seeds. Put the sriracha mayonnaise into sauce pots to serve on the side.

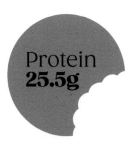

Protein
25.5g

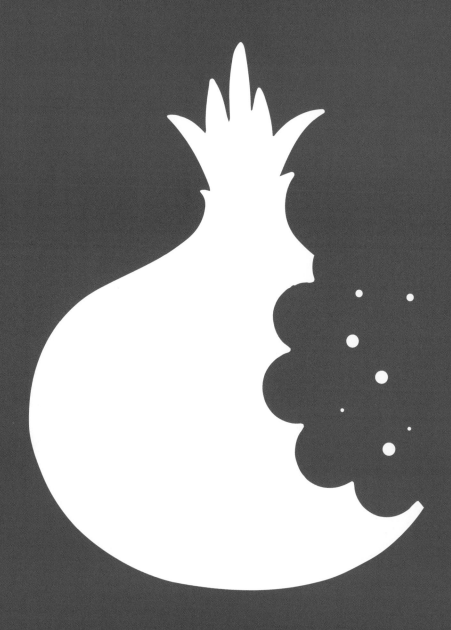

Set & Forget
Slow Cooks

Slow-cooker Chipotle Beef

Super easy to make and customizable into a variety of different dishes, this slow-cooker chipotle beef might just be a perfect meal prep recipe. The flavour of the beef is unmatched and, after 4 hours of slow cooking, the beef literally falls apart in your hands. Use this to make tacos, burritos or a rice bowl.

1kg braising steak (not diced)
1 tbsp unsalted butter
2 bay leaves
salt and pepper

For the chipotle sauce

400ml hot beef stock
2 tbsp ground cumin
2–3 tbsp chipotle paste
   (depending on how spicy
   you want it)
2 tbsp dried oregano
½ tbsp smoked paprika
1 tbsp onion granules
juice of 1 lime
4 cloves of garlic, peeled
½ tsp salt
2 tbsp apple cider vinegar

To serve as a rice bowl

125g cooked rice
2 tbsp pico de gallo or salsa
2 tbsp guacamole
1 tbsp soured cream
fresh coriander, chopped

To serve as a burrito

1 tortilla wrap
75g cooked rice
1 tbsp soured cream
Cheddar cheese, grated
fresh coriander, chopped

To serve as tacos

2 mini tortilla wraps
10g Cheddar or mozzarella
   cheese, grated or shredded
1 tbsp chopped red onion
1 tsp groundnut oil, for frying (or
   bake the tacos in the oven)
salsa
handful of coriander leaves

1. First, make the chipotle sauce. Combine all the ingredients in a food processor or blender and blend until smooth.

2. Season the steak liberally with salt and pepper, then heat the butter in a cast-iron or heavy-based frying pan over a high heat until smoking hot. Sear the steak for 3–4 minutes on each side, then transfer to a slow cooker. Pour the sauce over the steak and add the bay leaves. Cover with the lid, then cook on High for 4–6 hours, or until you can pull the beef apart using two forks. Once cooked, transfer the beef to a bowl and shred the beef with two forks. Spoon some of the sauce left in the slow cooker over the beef.

3. To serve the beef as a rice bowl, pile it into a bowl with the rice, pico de gallo or salsa, guacamole and soured cream, then top with the coriander. Alternatively, wrap it up into a burrito with some rice, soured cream, Cheddar and coriander. Or, pack it into some delicious tacos. Add the beef, Cheddar or mozzarella and onion to the mini tortillas, then fold over and fry in a little oil until crispy. Alternatively, bake or air fry the tacos. Store the slow-cooked beef in airtight containers in the fridge for up to 3 days.

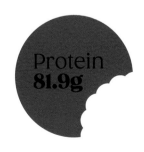

Protein
81.9g

Serves: **4**   Prep time: **5 mins**   Cook time: **4-6 hrs**

With rice: Cals: **698**   Carbs: **43.3g**   Protein: **78.8g**   Fat: **24.6g**

As a burrito: Cals: **818**   Carbs: **60.9g**   Protein: **84.5g**   Fat: **28.3g**

As tacos: Cals: **726**   Carbs: **35.9g**   Protein: **81.9g**   Fat: **29.7g**

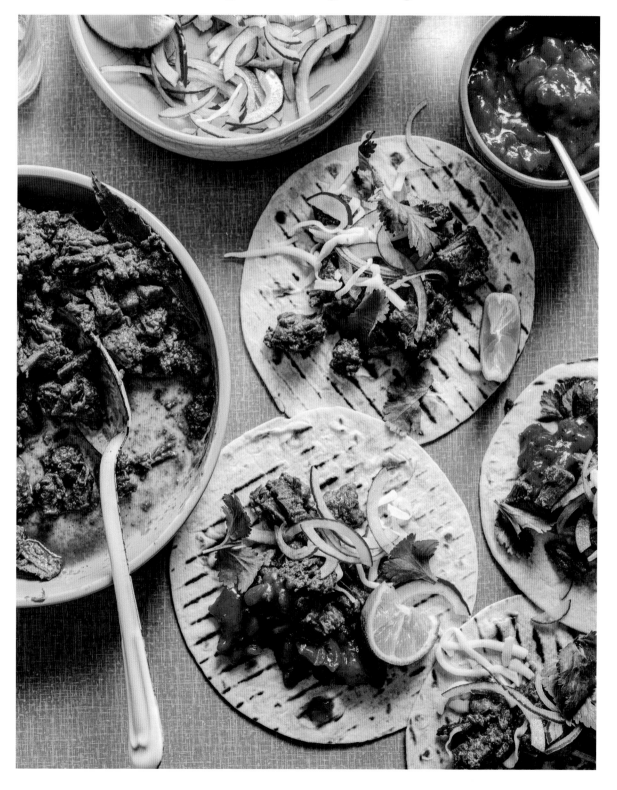

Slow-cooker Sweet Potato Shepherd's Pie

This is my twist on a home-comfort classic and it couldn't be easier to make. Just slow cook the beef mince filling for 4 hours until your home is filled with wonderfully comforting aromas, then top with sweet potato mash. This is healthy, high-protein cooking that will please a household or serve as a delightful packed lunch.

1 onion, finely chopped

2 carrots, peeled and finely chopped

2 sticks of celery, finely chopped

1 clove of garlic, peeled and crushed

2 tbsp Worcestershire sauce

500g lean beef mince (5% fat)

200ml hot beef stock

1 tbsp cornflour

1 x 400g tin of chopped tomatoes

1 tbsp balsamic vinegar

3 tbsp tomato purée

½ tbsp dried or fresh thyme

½ tbsp dried or fresh rosemary

salt and freshly ground black pepper

For the sweet potato mash topping

900g sweet potatoes, peeled and roughly chopped

1 tbsp unsalted butter

1 clove of garlic, peeled and crushed

50 g reduced-fat Cheddar cheese, grated

To serve

100g sliced kale, steamed

1. Put all the ingredients into a slow cooker, stir well, season and cook on High for 4 hours.

2. Meanwhile, bring a large saucepan of water to the boil and cook the sweet potatoes for 15 minutes until fork-tender, then drain and transfer to a large bowl. Add the butter, garlic, salt and pepper and mash until smooth.

3. Transfer the beef filling to a baking dish and top with the sweet potato mash. Sprinkle over the Cheddar, then place under a hot grill for 5–10 minutes until the cheese is melted and bubbling.

4. Divide among airtight containers and add the steamed kale, then store in the fridge for up to 4 days.

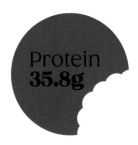

Protein
35.8g

Serves: **4**   Prep time: **10 mins**   Cook time: **4 hrs 10 mins**

Cals: **498**   Carbs: **66.7g**   Protein: **35.8g**   Fat: **11.2g**

9 780241 694015

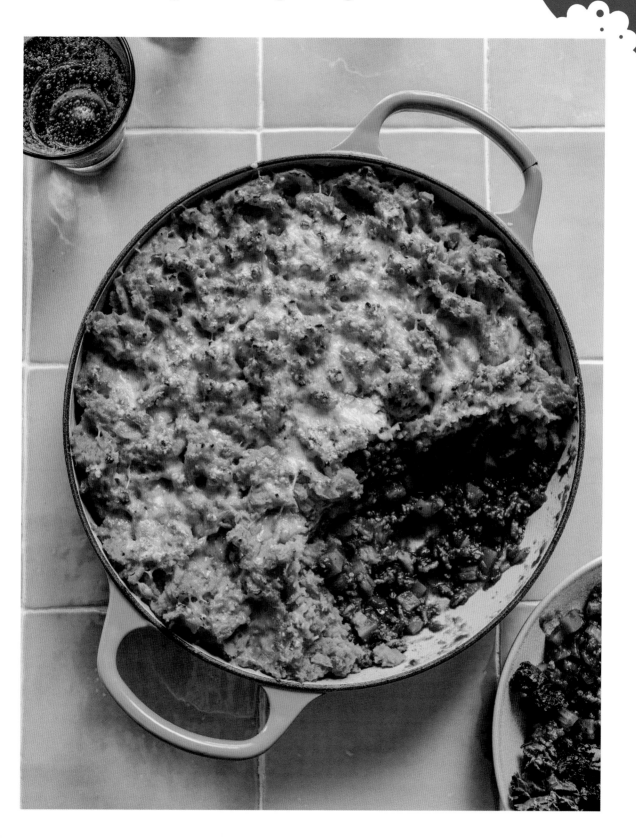

Serves: **4**   Prep time: **5 mins**   Cook time: **4 hrs**
Cals: **760**   Carbs: **76g**   Protein: **82.4g**   Fat: **16.2g**

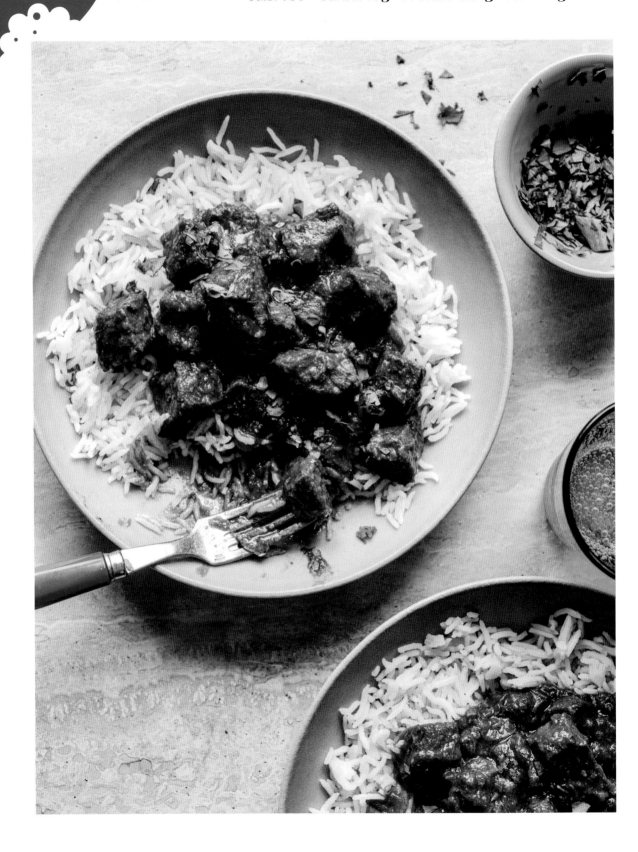

Slow-cooker Beef Curry

Curries are one of the best things you can make in a slow cooker and this rich beef recipe is no exception. All you need is a handful of ingredients, then chuck them into your slow cooker, cover and leave to stew for 4 hours. The result is a wonderfully flavourful curry that is healthy, high in protein and perfect for meal prepping.

800g braising steak, diced
2 onions, roughly chopped
4 cloves of garlic, peeled
   and grated
20g fresh ginger, peeled
   and grated
2 tbsp mild curry paste
1 tbsp mango chutney
1 tsp ground turmeric
½ tsp chilli powder
5 cardamom pods
1 x 400g tin of chopped tomatoes
250ml beef stock
a small bunch of fresh coriander,
   finely chopped, plus extra to
   serve
300g basmati rice

1. Put all the ingredients, except the rice, into a slow cooker, stir to combine and cook on High for 4 hours.

2. Meanwhile, bring a large saucepan of water to the boil and cook the rice according to the packet instructions, then drain.

3. Transfer the rice and curry to airtight containers, sprinkle with extra coriander and store in the fridge for up to 4 days.

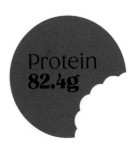

Protein
82.4g

9 780241 694046

Serves: **4**   Prep time: **5 mins**   Cook time: **3 hrs 30 mins**

Cals: **696**   Carbs: **92.6g**   Protein: **47g**   Fat: **16.6g**

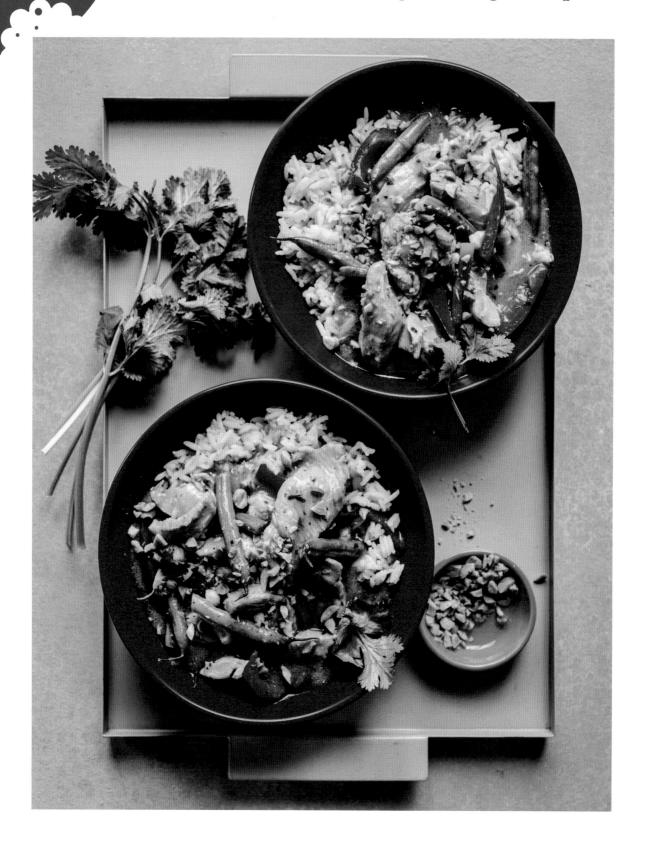

Slow-cooker Thai Green Curry

Thai green curry is full of vibrant, aromatic flavours and cooking it in a slow cooker only enhances those elements, while also being healthy and light in calories. I've provided two options for the protein source (chicken or prawns) and the carbohydrate source (rice or noodles). It's a super flexible recipe, so feel free to experiment for yourself by adding different vegetables or other protein sources like tofu.

2 tbsp Thai green curry paste
1 tbsp dark soy sauce
1 tbsp fish sauce
1 large shallot, peeled and
  finely chopped
500g chicken breast, thinly sliced,
  or 350g raw, peeled king prawns
150ml hot chicken stock
2 red peppers, sliced
200g green beans, topped
  and tailed
10g fresh ginger, peeled and
  thinly sliced
1 red chilli, thinly sliced
a small bunch of fresh coriander,
  finely chopped.
1 x 400ml tin of reduced-fat
  coconut milk
100ml boiling water

To serve
600g cooked jasmine rice or
  straight-to-wok egg noodles
fresh coriander, leaves picked
40g roasted peanuts, chopped

1. Put the curry paste, soy sauce, fish sauce, shallot, chicken (if using king prawns instead, add these later) and stock into a slow cooker, stir to combine, then cook on High for 3 hours.

2. After this time, add the king prawns, if using, red pepper, green beans, ginger, chilli, coriander, coconut milk and boiling water. Stir to combine, then cook on High for a further 30 minutes. If serving the curry with noodles, add them to the slow cooker for the final 5 minutes of cooking time.

3. Transfer the curry (and rice, if using) to airtight containers, garnish with the coriander and chopped peanuts, then store in the fridge for up to 4 days.

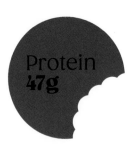

Protein
47g

Slow-cooker Steak Pie

Is there anything more comforting than a steak pie? Is there anything easier than a slow-cooker recipe? The answer to both of those questions is no by the way! And for those reasons, I felt like I had to include this recipe in my book. A rich beef filling, stewed until falling apart, is topped with golden and crispy puff pastry. Feel free to swap out the puff pastry for a mashed potato topping if you prefer.

800g stewing steak, diced
600ml beef stock
1 onion, thinly sliced
2 cloves of garlic, peeled and
   thinly sliced
2 carrots, chopped
2 sticks of celery, finely chopped
1 tbsp tomato purée
2 tbsp Worcestershire sauce
2 sprigs of fresh thyme, leaves
   chopped
1 x 320g sheet of puff pastry
1 egg, beaten
plain flour, for dusting
steamed kale, to serve

1. Put all the ingredients, except the pastry, egg, flour and kale, into a slow cooker. Stir to combine, then cook on High for 4 hours, stirring occasionally.

2. When the filling has almost finished cooking, preheat the oven to 200°C (180°C fan/400°F/Gas 6).

3. Transfer the pie filling to a large baking dish, then roll out the pastry on a lightly floured surface and place on top. Cut off any excess pastry around the edges and press the pastry lightly into the pie filling. Brush the beaten egg over the pastry. Bake in the oven for 20 minutes until crisp and golden. Remove from the oven and allow to cool slightly.

4. Cut the pie into four pieces, then transfer to airtight containers with the kale. Store in the fridge for up to 4 days.

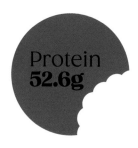

Protein
52.6g

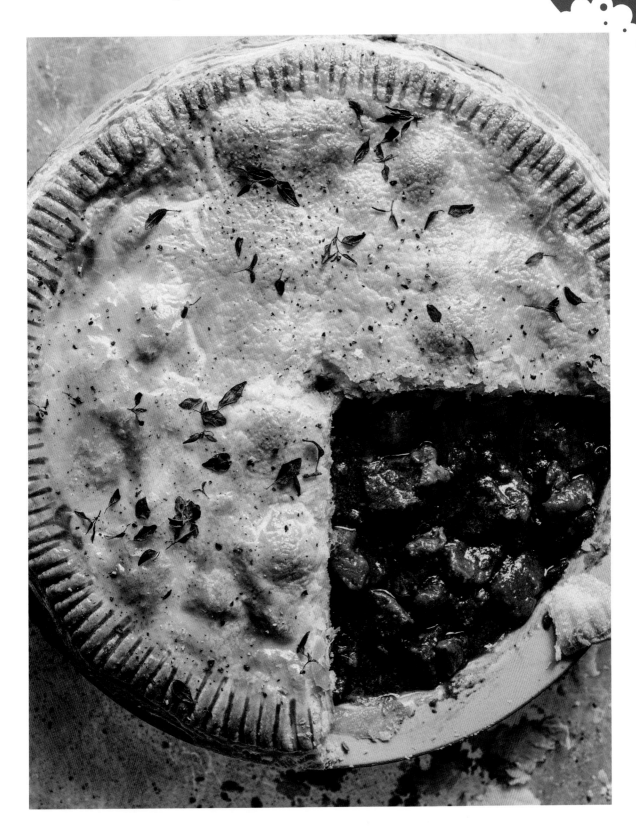

Slow-cooker Baked Bean Chilli

Baked beans in a chilli?! Trust me, you need to try this super-nutritious and tasty baked bean chilli. Beans are full of antioxidants, high in fibre and an amazing plant-based source of protein. The tomato sauce from the baked beans adds another level of sweetness and richness to this recipe and it couldn't be any simpler to make – all you need to do is fry the onion and throw it all into a slow cooker and let the wonderful flavours fuse together. Best served hot.

1 tbsp extra virgin olive oil
1 onion, thinly sliced
1 stick of celery, finely chopped
3 peppers (a mixture of colours), roughly chopped
1 x 400g tin of chopped tomatoes
1 x 400g tin of kidney beans, drained
1 x 400g tin of black beans, drained
2 x 415g tins of baked beans
1 tbsp chipotle paste
150ml vegetable stock
250g passata
1 tsp garlic granules
½ tbsp ground cumin
½ tbsp smoked paprika
600g cooked basmati rice, to serve
Cheddar cheese, grated, to serve

1. Heat the olive oil in a frying pan over a low heat and cook the onion for 10 minutes, stirring regularly, then transfer to a slow cooker along with all the other ingredients. Stir well, then cook on High for 4 hours.

2. Transfer to airtight containers with the basmati rice and Cheddar and store in the fridge for up to 4 days.

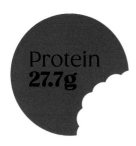

Protein
27.7g

Serves: **4**   Prep time: **5 mins**   Cook time: **4 hrs**
Cals: **568**   Carbs: **91.7g**   Protein: **27.7g**   Fat: **9.3g**

175

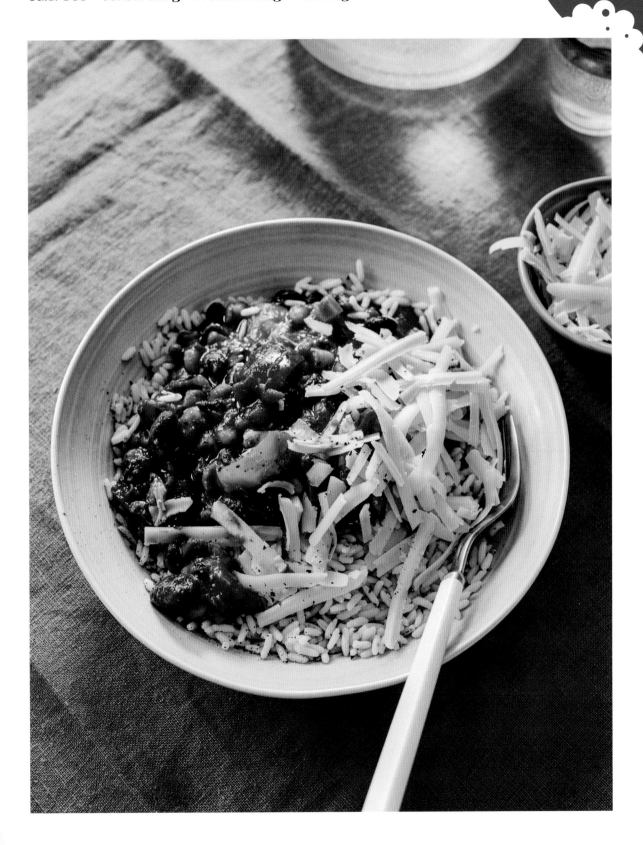

Serves: **4**   Prep time: **5 mins**   Cook time: **3 hrs 30 mins**

Cals: **567**   Carbs: **67.6g**   Protein: **48.6g**   Fat: **10.7g**

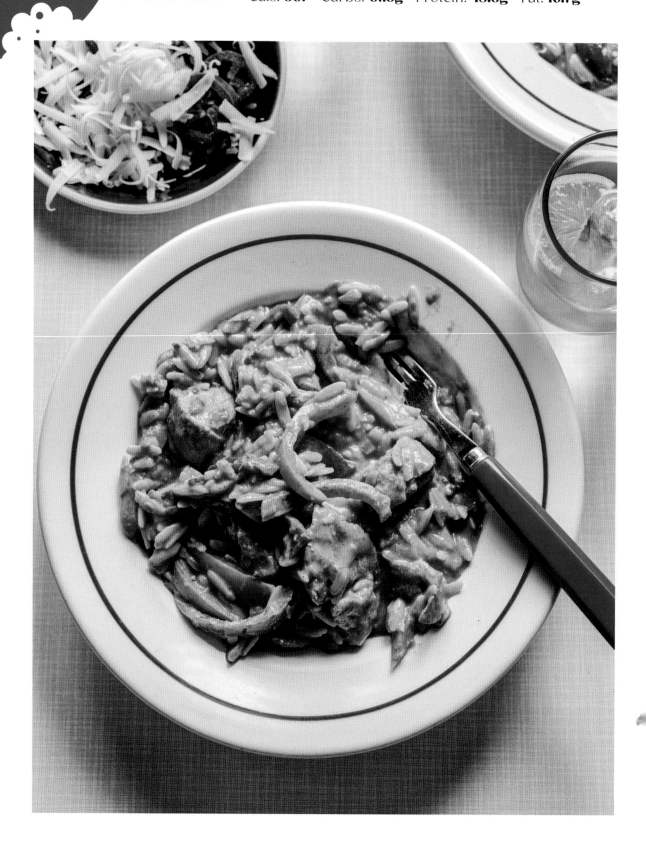

Slow-cooker Fajita Orzotto

This is called an 'orzotto' because it is cooked risotto-style. You cook the chicken and vegetables with the tomatoes, chicken stock and fajita seasoning, creating an amazingly tasty sauce, then add the orzo and cream and cook slowly until you are left with a heavenly creamy orzo risotto. This is all cooked in the slow cooker, making it super fuss-free, and it's light in calories and high in protein, too. Be careful not to overcook the orzo, as it will become stodgy, and transfer to your meal prep containers as quickly as you can.

500g chicken breast, diced
1 onion, finely chopped
3 cloves of garlic, peeled
  and crushed
1 x 400g tin of chopped tomatoes
4 tbsp Fajita Seasoning (see
  page 158 or use shop-bought)
700ml chicken stock
2 tbsp tomato purée
2 fresh jalapeños, thinly sliced (and
  deseeded depending on spice
  preference)
1 green pepper, sliced
1 orange pepper, sliced
2 roasted peppers (from a jar),
  drained, or 1 red pepper, sliced
250g orzo
125ml single cream
30g reduced-fat Cheddar cheese,
  grated
salt and freshly ground
  black pepper

1. Put the chicken, onion, garlic, chopped tomatoes, fajita seasoning and 200ml of the chicken stock into a slow cooker, stir to combine, then cook on High for 3 hours, stirring occasionally.

2. Add the tomato purée, jalapeños, peppers, orzo and remaining chicken stock and cook on High for 30 minutes.

3. Stir in the single cream, check and adjust the seasoning, then sprinkle over the grated Cheddar and cover until the cheese has completely melted.

4. Divide among airtight containers and store in the fridge for up to 4 days.

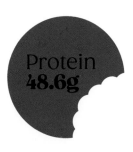

Protein
48.6g

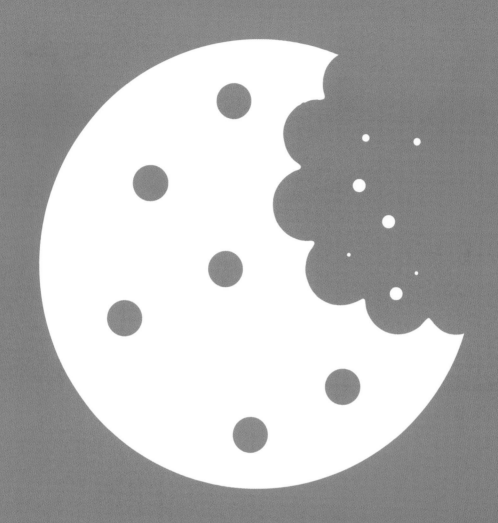

Protein
Puds

Biscoff Protein Truffles

Just five ingredients are needed to make a batch of these utterly delicious Biscoff protein truffles. They are the perfect treat to keep in the fridge, ready to be called upon whenever you feel like indulging that sweet tooth.

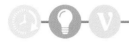

150g Biscoff biscuits, plus extra crumbs for sprinkling
100g light cream cheese
2 tbsp Biscoff spread
50g vanilla protein powder
150g white chocolate, roughly chopped
sea salt (optional)

1. Put the biscuits into a food processor and pulse to a fine crumb. Add the cream cheese, 1 tablespoon of the Biscoff spread and the vanilla protein powder and pulse again until you have a sticky dough.

2. Scrape the mixture out onto a clean surface and divide it into 16 evenly sized balls (roughly 20–25g per ball). Place the balls on a baking tray lined with baking paper and chill in the fridge or freezer for 15–30 minutes until firm.

3. Put the white chocolate into a bowl and microwave on high for 20 second intervals until completely melted.

4. Dip each chilled truffle in the chocolate, using a fork to coat them all over, then transfer back to the lined baking tray.

5. Melt the remaining tablespoon of Biscoff spread in the microwave, then drizzle over the truffles to decorate. Top with a sprinkle of biscuit crumbs.

6. Leave to set (you can speed up this process by refrigerating the truffles), then transfer to an airtight container and store in the fridge for up to 4 days.

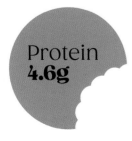

Protein
4.6g

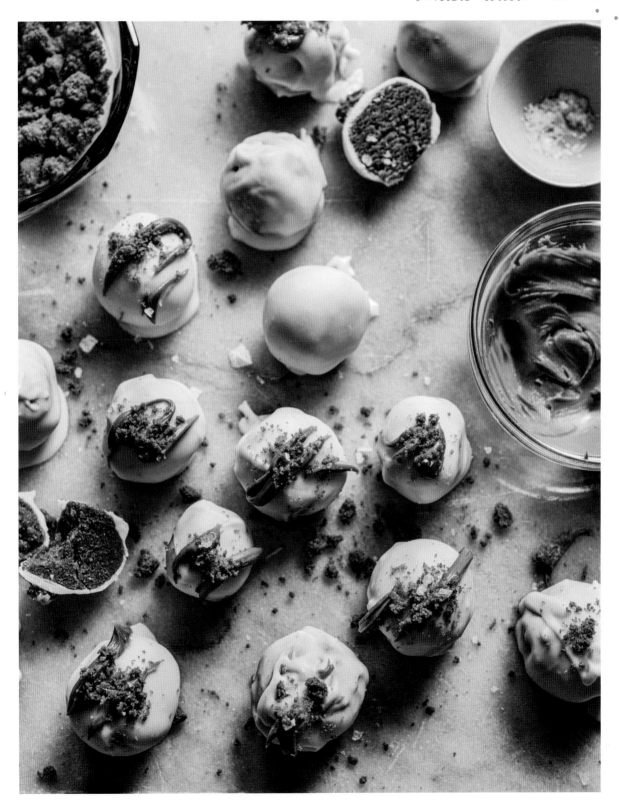

Cookie Dough Bites

There is no butter and no flour in these cookie dough bites – they're just high in protein and absolutely delicious. These are intended to be eaten as an energizing snack or moreish after-dinner sweet treat.

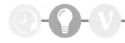

70g oat flour
40g ground almonds
50g vanilla protein powder
150g smooth natural peanut butter
1 tbsp coconut oil, melted
1 tsp vanilla extract
25g milk chocolate chips, for cookie dough
175g milk chocolate chips, to coat each bite

1. In a large bowl or food processor, combine the oat flour, ground almonds and protein powder. Stir or pulse to mix. Add the peanut butter, coconut oil and vanilla extract and mix or pulse together until you have a mixture that resembles cookie dough. Transfer to a bowl, if necessary, and fold in the milk chocolate chips.

2. Scrape the mixture out onto a clean surface and divide it into 15 evenly sized balls. Place the balls on a baking tray lined with baking paper and chill in the fridge or freezer for 1 hour until firm.

3. Put the remaining milk chocolate chips into a bowl and microwave on high for 30 second intervals until completely melted.

4. Dip each chilled cookie dough bite in the chocolate, using a fork to coat them all over, then transfer back to the lined baking tray.

5. Leave to set (you can speed up this process by refrigerating the cookie dough bites), then transfer to an airtight container and store in the fridge for up to 4 days.

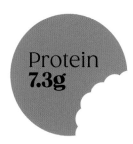

Protein
7.3g

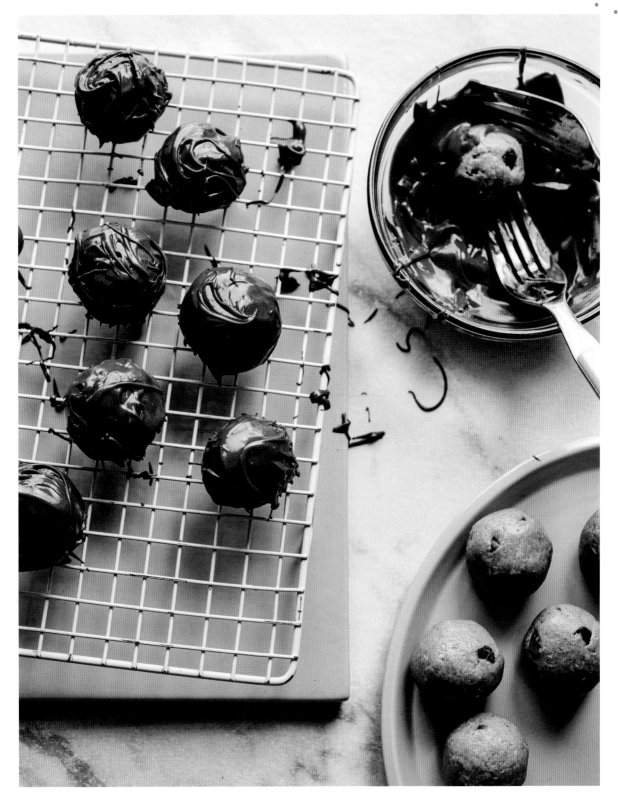

Makes: **6**   Prep time: **10 mins**   Cook time: **10 mins**

Cals: **189**   Carbs: **19.6g**   Protein: **20.7g**   Fat: **3.5g**

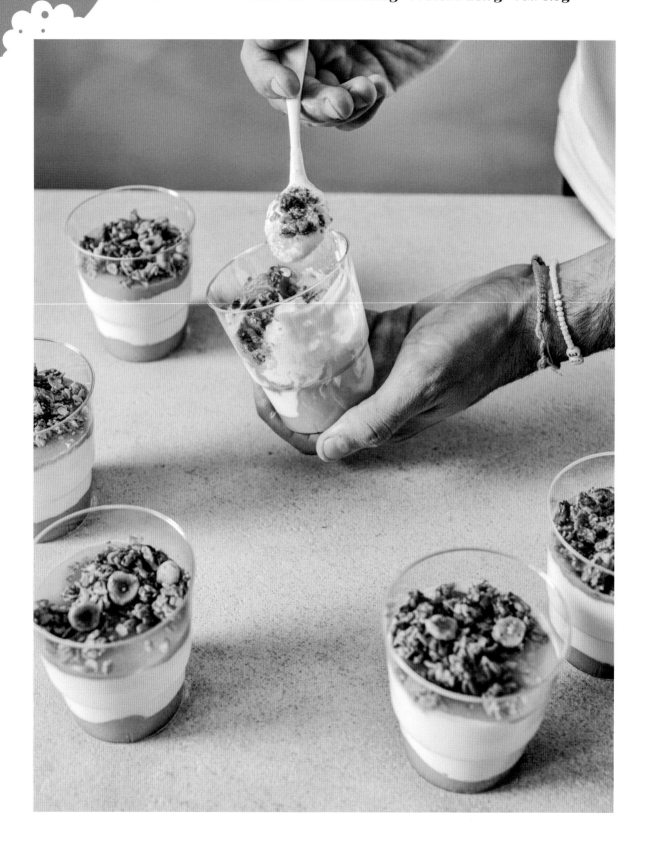

Mango Protein Yoghurts

Yoghurt pots are a staple of almost any high street café or lunch spot, but what if I told you that you could save yourself a lot of money and increase your daily protein intake by making these banging mango protein pots at home? The simple combination of vanilla protein powder and Greek yoghurt is something I have been using as a dessert for years, and it's accompanied perfectly by a sweet and tangy mango compote. The perfect healthy and high-protein pudding.

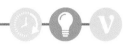

600g mango chunks
1 tbsp maple syrup
juice of ½ lemon
3 scoops of vanilla protein powder
500g fat-free Greek yoghurt
40g granola, to serve

1. Put the mango, maple syrup, lemon juice and 2 tablespoons water in a saucepan over a medium heat and simmer for 5–7 minutes until the mango starts to break down, stirring occasionally to make sure it's not sticking. Reduce the heat to low, add a splash more water if it needs it, and cook for a further 5 minutes, stirring regularly, until soft and jammy. Transfer to a blender or food processor and blend until smooth.

2. In a large bowl, mix together the vanilla protein powder and yoghurt until fully combined, with no lumps.

3. Add a splash of water to the mango compote to loosen it if needed. Divide roughly half the mixture among six yoghurt pots or small glasses, then add the protein yoghurt mixture. Top with the remaining mango compote and sprinkle over the granola to finish. Store in the fridge for up to 5 days.

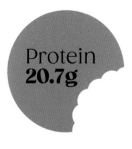

Protein
20.7g

9 780241 694121

Serves: **4**   Prep time: **5 mins**

Cals: **229**   Carbs: **14.4g**   Protein: **23.8g**   Fat: **8.6g**

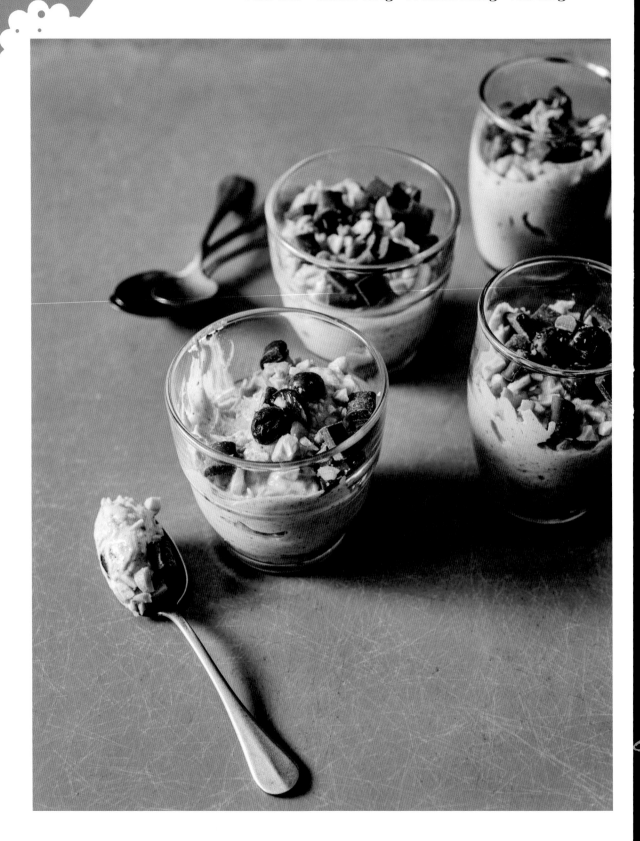

Peanut Butter Protein Pots

These joyous little puddings are packed full of protein and require almost zero effort to make. All you need to do is combine the yoghurt, protein powder, peanut butter and honey to create a deliciously creamy, smooth, sweet and nutty pudding, then just fold in some fresh blueberries and serve – simple and delicious.

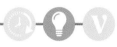

350g fat-free Greek yoghurt
50g vanilla protein powder
3 tbsp smooth natural
  peanut butter
2 tbsp runny honey
50g blueberries
15g blanched peanuts, chopped,
  to garnish

1. In a large bowl, combine the yoghurt, protein powder, peanut butter and honey. Stir until smooth with no lumps, then fold in the blueberries, reserving some to garnish.

2. Divide the mixture among four small airtight containers and garnish with the chopped peanuts and blueberries. These will keep in the fridge for up to 4 days.

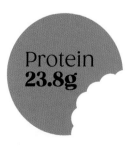

Protein
23.8g

Serves: **4**   Prep time: **10 mins**   Cook time: **5 mins**
Cals: **368**   Carbs: **23.5g**   Protein: **7.9g**   Fat: **26.7g**

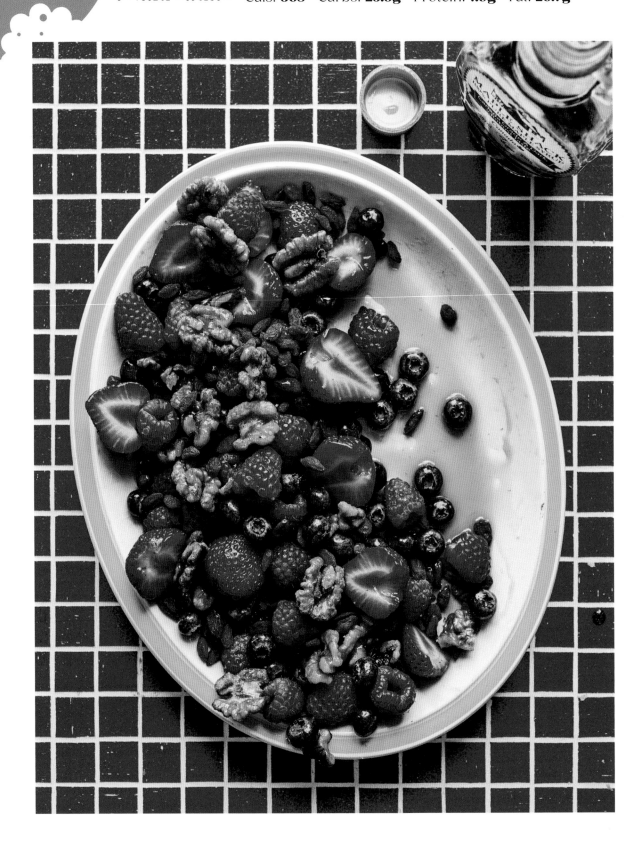

Candied Walnut Fruit Salad

If you always end up with mouldy fruit sat at the back of the fridge or struggle to eat enough fruit (like me), then you need to try this fruit salad. It's an easy and delicious way to pack more fruit into your diet, and meal preps perfectly. The candied walnuts are delicious, sweet and crunchy and match this refreshing fruit salad dreamily. Use this as a healthy, on-the-go snack or dessert.

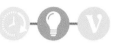

150g walnut halves
2–3 tbsp maple syrup, plus extra
   if desired
150g strawberries, hulled and
   halved
150g blueberries
150g raspberries
30g goji berries
a squeeze of lime juice

1. Preheat the oven to 180°C (160°C fan/350°F/Gas 4) and line a baking tray with baking paper.

2. Put the walnuts into a large bowl with the maple syrup and stir to coat. Transfer to the prepared baking tray and bake in the oven for 5–6 minutes until glossy and crisp. Remove from the oven and leave to cool.

3. Meanwhile, combine the strawberries, blueberries, raspberries and goji berries in a large bowl, then add the lime juice and another tablespoon of maple syrup, if you like. Stir to combine.

4. Transfer the fruit salad to a large airtight container and store in the fridge for 3–4 days. If possible, store the candied walnuts in a separate airtight container to help them keep their texture and serve on top of the fruit salad before eating.

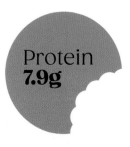

Protein
7.9g

Oreo Protein Brownies

I have been making these ridiculously straightforward Oreo protein brownies for years and they always go down a treat in my household. All you need are five ingredients! I skip the butter and sugar and use bananas and peanut butter instead to achieve a naturally sweet and rich, gooey chocolate brownie with bits of broken up Oreo throughout.

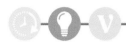

3 overripe bananas
250g smooth natural peanut butter
50g vanilla protein powder
3 tbsp cocoa powder
8 Oreos

1. Preheat the oven to 180°C (160°C fan/350°F/Gas 4) and line a loaf tin or baking tray with baking paper.

2. Mash the bananas in a bowl, then stir in the peanut butter, protein powder and cocoa powder until you are left with a brownie batter. Break up half the Oreos and fold into the batter.

3. Transfer the mixture to the prepared loaf tin, then break up the remaining Oreos and sprinkle over the top.

4. Bake in the oven for 15 minutes, then remove from the oven and allow to cool for 10–15 minutes before slicing into 10 brownies. This will keep in the fridge for up to 4 days.

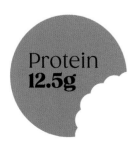

Protein
12.5g

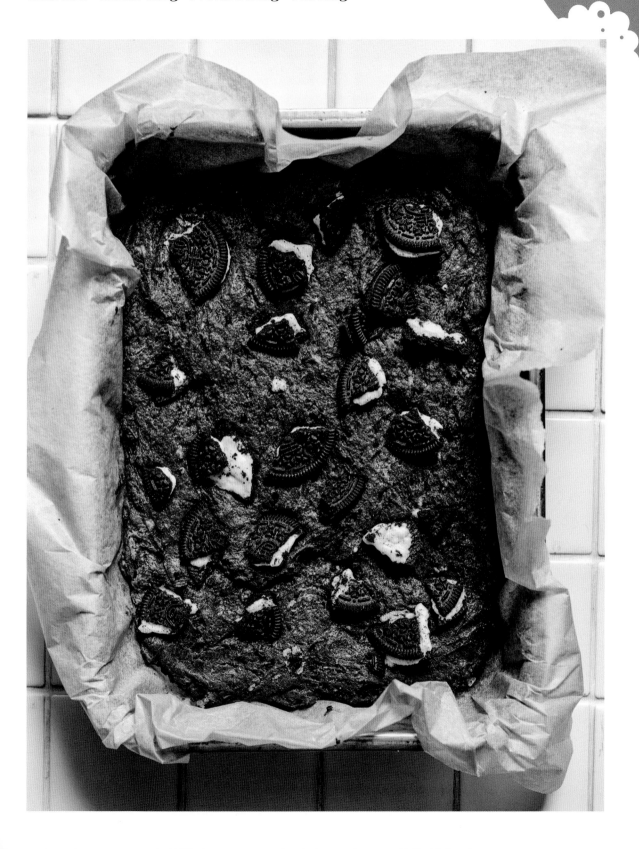

Serves: **4**   Prep time: **5 mins**   Cook time: **20 mins**
Cals: **413**   Carbs: **65.9g**   Protein: **22.2g**   Fat: **8.5g**

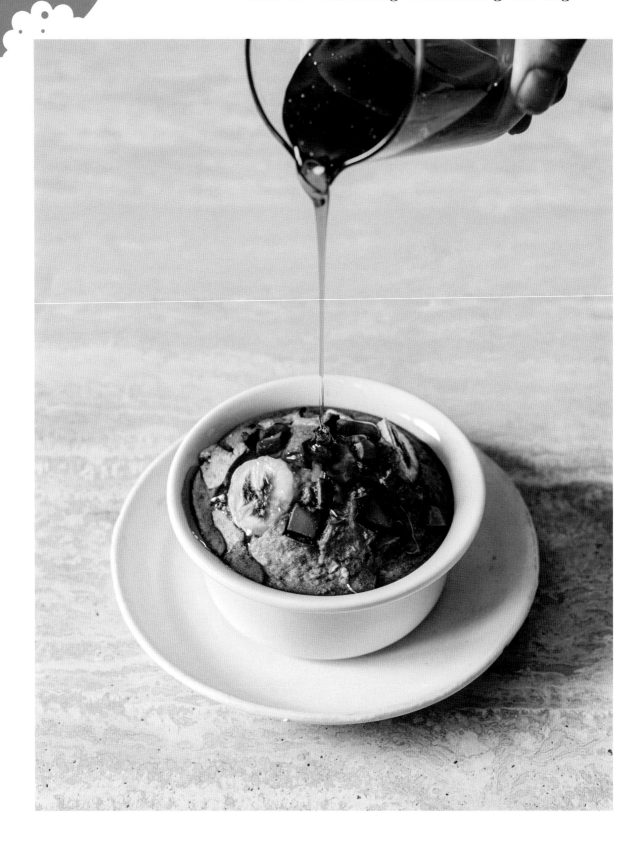

Banana Bread Baked Oats

A banging, high-protein baked oats recipe that comes out of the oven smelling and tasting just like banana bread! Rather than baking these in four separate baking dishes, you could also bake them in one large dish and slice it up into four servings. These are perfect served with a drizzle of maple syrup.

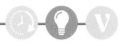

4 bananas
160g rolled oats
1 tbsp maple syrup, plus extra to serve
1 tsp ground cinnamon
75g vanilla protein powder
2 tsp baking powder
300ml almond milk
30g milk chocolate chips

1. Preheat the oven to 180°C (160°C fan/350°F/Gas 4).

2. Put three of the bananas, the oats, maple syrup, cinnamon, protein powder, baking powder and milk into a blender and blend until smooth. Pour the mixture into four wide ramekins or small baking dishes.

3. Slice the remaining banana and arrange on top, then sprinkle over the chocolate chips.

4. Bake in the oven for 20 minutes.

5. Transfer to airtight containers and keep in the fridge for up to 4 days. Add a drizzle of maple syrup before serving, if you wish.

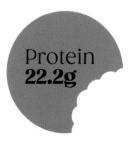

Protein
22.2g

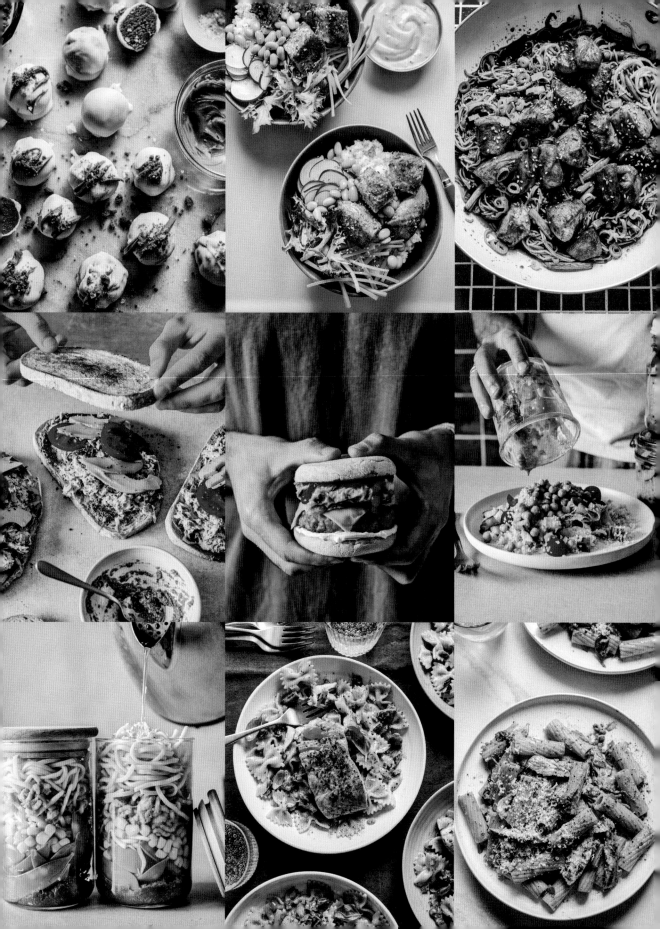

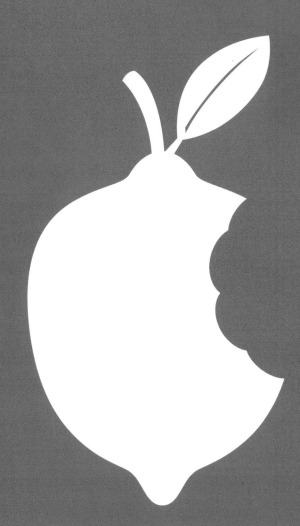

Index

Index

D

E

F

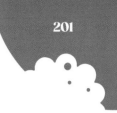

R

S

V

W

y

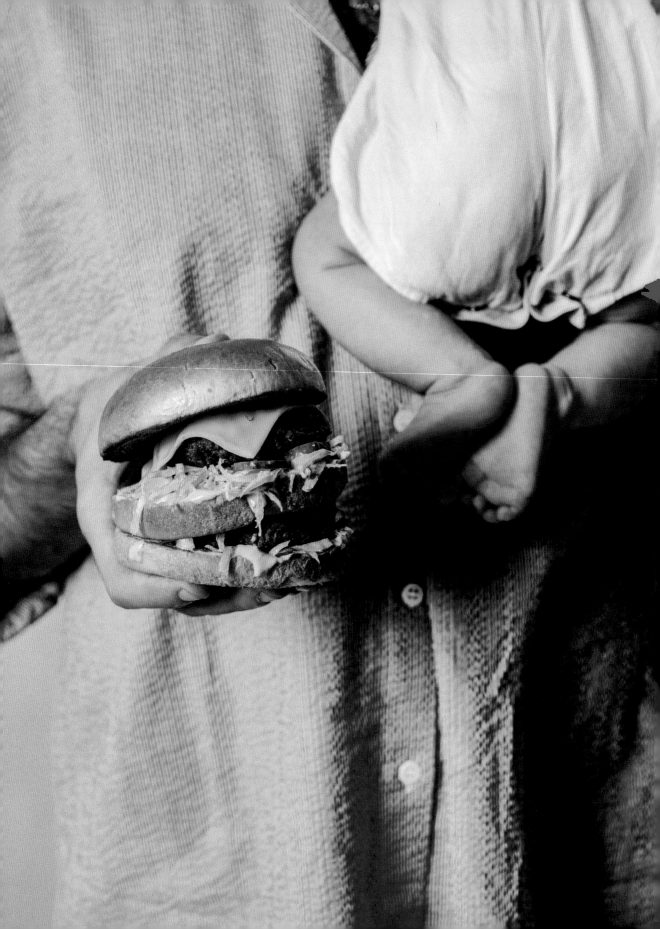

Thanks . . .

There are a lot more people than just me who have made this book a reality, and I'm so unbelievably grateful for their support and guidance throughout the journey, so let me shout them out.

Firstly, I need to mention and give the biggest thank you to my right-hand man and best friend, Karl. He films, edits, tastes (and critiques) everything that you see on The Good Bite and the page wouldn't be what it is today without him. He also held down the fort on all our platforms when I was busy developing the recipes for this book, so thank you, Karl!

Thank you to my beautiful wife, Megan, who has supported me since day one of my journey as a food creator. Our daughter, Winnie, was born two weeks before the final deadline for this book, so as you can imagine, things got a bit hectic. Megan was selfless and supported me unwaveringly throughout the busy schedule, so thank you so much from the bottom of my heart.

Thank you to Oscar, who landed me this amazing book deal, and Babz, Eloise and the whole team at Gleam, who have pushed me in a direction I could only dream of.

Thank you to Dan, Aggie and Michael Joseph, firstly for giving me this incredible opportunity but also for being so amazing to work with. Thank you to my copy-editor, Lucy, and to Georgie, who made the book look absolutely unreal.

Thank you to Max and Liz – working with you was a 'pinch myself' moment and every single picture looks incredible. Thank you, too, to Rosie, Troy, Jess and Eyder for making the food look so delicious.

And, of course, thank you to you guys, the readers. It still doesn't seem real that I have my own cookbook published, but I could not be happier with the end result. If you're a follower of me or The Good Bite, then thank you, because this book wouldn't have happened without you. Or, if you've just picked up this book in a shop and have never heard of me, then thank you as well! I hope you love the recipes in this book as much as I do, and I really hope they help you live a healthier and happier life.

PENGUIN MICHAEL JOSEPH

UK | USA | Canada | Ireland | Australia
India | New Zealand | South Africa

Penguin Michael Joseph is part of the Penguin Random House group of companies
whose addresses can be found at global.penguinrandomhouse.com

Penguin Random House UK, One Embassy Gardens,
8 Viaduct Gardens, London SW11 7BW

penguin.co.uk

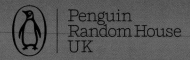

First published 2023
006

Set in Gazpacho and Sofia Pro
Design by Georgie Hewitt
Food styling by Rosie Reynolds and Troy Willis
Colour reproduction by AltaImage Ltd
Printed and bound in Germany by Mohn Media

The authorized representative in the EEA is Penguin Random House Ireland,
Morrison Chambers, 32 Nassau Street, Dublin D02 YH68

A CIP catalogue record for this book is available from the British Library

ISBN: 978-0-241-67561-8

Penguin Random House is committed to a sustainable future
for our business, our readers and our planet. This book is made from
Forest Stewardship Council® certified paper.

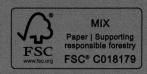